World Religions for Healthcare Professionals

Religious beliefs and customs can significantly shape patients' and professionals' attitudes toward, and expectations of, healthcare, as well as their wishes and personal boundaries regarding such daily matters as dress, diet, prayer, and touch. Undoubtedly, the sensitivity with which clinicians communicate with patients and make decisions regarding appropriate medical intervention can be greatly increased by an understanding of religious as well as other forms of cultural diversity.

This second edition of a popular and established text offers healthcare students and professionals a clear and concise overview of health beliefs and practices in world religions, including Hinduism, Buddhism, Jainism, Confucianism, Taoism, Sikhism, Islam, Judaism, and Christianity. Adopting a consistent structure, each chapter considers the demographic profile of the community, the religion's historical development, and key beliefs and practices, including views regarding health and sickness, death, and dying. Each chapter also ends with a useful checklist of advice on what to do and what to avoid, along with recommendations for further reading, both online and in print form.

The book's clear and consistent style ensures that readers with little background knowledge can find the information they need and assimilate it easily. A brand new chapter on applications and a set of new case studies illustrating issues in clinical practice enhance this wide-ranging book's value to students and practitioners alike.

Siroj Sorajjakool has studied and taught world religions in university and healthcare settings for over 25 years. He is a professor in the School of Religion at Loma Linda University.

Mark F. Carr has studied and taught in the areas of religion, theology, ethics, and bioethics for over 20 years. He holds a clinical ethics and administrative position at Providence Health and Services, Alaska.

Ernest J. Bursey has studied and taught in the areas of religion, theology, New Testament, and healthcare for over 40 years. He teaches on these topics at the Adventist University of Healthcare Sciences.

World Religions for Healthcare Professionals

Second edition edited by
Siroj Sorajjakool, Mark F. Carr,
and Ernest J. Bursey

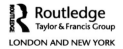

LONDON AND NEW YORK

Second edition published 2017
by Routledge
2 Park Square, Milton Park, Abingdon, Oxon OX14 4RN

and by Routledge
711 Third Avenue, New York, NY 10017

Routledge is an imprint of the Taylor & Francis Group, an informa business

© 2017 Siroj Sorajjakool, Mark F. Carr, and Ernest J. Bursey

First edition published by Routledge 2009.

British Library Cataloguing in Publication Data
A catalogue record for this book is available from the British Library

Library of Congress Cataloging in Publication Data
Names: Sorajjakool, Siroj, editor. | Carr, Mark F., editor. | Bursey,
Ernest J., editor.
Title: World religions for healthcare professionals / [edited by] Siroj
Sorajjakool, Mark F. Carr, and Ernest J. Bursey.
Description: Second edition. | Abingdon, Oxon ; New York, NY :
Routledge, 2017. | Includes bibliographical references and index.
Identifiers: LCCN 2016043134| ISBN 9781138189133 (hbk.) |
ISBN 9781138189140 (pbk.) | ISBN 9781315641775 (ebk.)
Subjects: LCSH: Medicine–Religious aspects. | Religions. | Cults. |
MESH: Religion and Medicine | Spirituality | Cultural Competency |
Patient Care–psychology | Professional-Patient Relations
Classification: LCC BL65.M4 W67 2017 | NLM BL 65.M4 | DDC
201/.661–dc23
LC record available at https://lccn.loc.gov/2016043134

ISBN: 978-1-138-18913-3 (hbk)
ISBN: 978-1-138-18914-0 (pbk)
ISBN: 978-1-315-64177-5 (ebk)

Typeset in Sabon
by Wearset Ltd, Boldon, Tyne and Wear

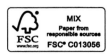

MIX
Paper from
responsible sources
FSC
www.fsc.org   FSC® C013056

Printed and bound in Great Britain by
TJ International Ltd, Padstow, Cornwall

Contents

vi *Contents*

Contributors

Whitny Braun, PhD, is an assistant professor of ethics in the School of Religion at Loma Linda University as well as a clinical bioethicist and public health professional who specializes in the ethics of intercultural engagement in the healthcare setting. She is also a contributor to the *Huffington Post* and her work has been seen on the National Geographic Channel and heard on NPR. She was formerly the director of the Center for Jain Studies at Claremont School of Theology and has been active in the legal matter of the Jain death ritual of Sallekhanā before the Indian courts.

Ernest J. Bursey, PhD, is professor of religion in the department of Health and Biomedical Sciences at Adventist University of Health Sciences in Orlando, Florida. He received his doctoral degree from Yale University in the field of religious studies with a dissertation on exorcism in the Gospel of Matthew. He has had a long academic career at Walla Walla University where he served as dean of the School of Theology, and more recently at Adventist University of Health Sciences where he teaches undergraduate and graduate level courses in Spirituality and Healthcare, World Religions, Bioethics, and Biblical Studies.

Mark F. Carr, PhD, served as professor of ethics in the School of Religion at Loma Linda University and the theological co-director of the Center for Christian Bioethics at the same institution. He received his doctoral degree in religious ethics at the University of Virginia and wrote *Passionate Deliberation: Emotion, Temperance, and the Care Ethic in Clinical Moral Deliberation* (2001). After a brief time as chair of the Humanities and Social Sciences Department at Kettering College in Ohio, he now works in Anchorage, Alaska, where he serves as the region director of ethics for Providence Health and Services.

Carla Gober, PhD, is director of the Center for Spiritual Life and Wholeness, assistant vice president for spiritual life and an assistant professor at Loma Linda University School of Religion. She holds bachelor's degrees in nursing and religion and master's degrees in public health education and marriage and family studies. She has worked as a marriage and family counselor, a specialist in spiritual care and grief therapy, and a health educator. She completed her doctorate in religious studies from Emory University where her focus was in the area of attachment, memory, and meaning.

Roy Kim, MD, is a staff physician at Riverside-San Bernardino County (California) Indian Health, Inc. He graduated from Loma Linda University School of Medicine and completed his family medicine residency at Florida Hospital in Orlando. He went on to a faculty development fellowship at Emory University's department of family and preventive medicine, at which time he also received his master of public health degree from Emory's Rollins School of Public Health. He has worked with the World Health Organization in Kosovo treating the Roma, Ashkali, and Egyptian Gypsy population. He has also tended to patients in Africa, Asia, Eastern Europe, and South America.

Douglas Kohn, MAHL, is senior rabbi of Congregation Emanu El in San Bernardino, California. He received his graduate and rabbinic training at Hebrew Union College-Jewish Institute of Religion, culminating in his ordination in 1987. Prior to his current post, he served as the rabbi of Beth Tikvah Congregation in Hoffman Estate, Illinois, and assistant and associate rabbi in synagogues in Buffalo and Baltimore. He has also served as an adjunct instructor for Hilbert College in Hamburg, New York. He is the editor of *Life, Faith, and Cancer: Jewish Journeys through Diagnosis* (2008).

David R. Larson, DMin, PhD, is professor of religion at Loma Linda University School of Religion. His specialty is in ethics from a Christian perspective, with a particular focus on bioethics. At Loma Linda University, he helped found the Center for Christian Bioethics, which has grown to be an important resource in the discipline. He received his DMin degree from Claremont School of Theology and PhD degree from Claremont Graduate University. He edited *Abortion: Ethical Issues and Options* (1992) and co-edited *Christianity and Homosexuality: Some Seventh-day Adventist Perspectives* (2008).

Arvind Mandair, PhD, is endowed professor of Sikh studies at the University of Michigan at Ann Arbor where he holds the SBSC chair in Sikh studies. He received his PhD in chemistry from Aston University in Birmingham, United Kingdom, and PhD in philosophy/Sikh studies from the University of Warwick, also in the UK. He is the author of *Religion and the Specter of the West: Sikhism, India, Postcoloniality and the Politics of Translation* (Columbia University Press, 2009). He is the founding co-editor of the journal *Sikh Formations: Religion, Culture and Theory*, published by Routledge.

Hamid Mavani, PhD, is assistant professor of Islamic studies at Claremont Graduate University, School of Religion. He obtained his graduate degrees from McGill University and received theological training from the seminaries in Qum, Cairo, and Damascus. This has enabled him to be an active contributor in both the academic and community discourses. His primary fields of interest include Islamic legal reform, women and Shi'i law, Shi'i theology and political thought, Muslims in America, Qur'anic studies, and contemporary developments in the Muslim world.

Supaporn Naewbood, DrPH, is a lecturer in nursing at Narasuan University, Pitsanulok, Thailand, and a doctoral student in public health nursing at Mahidol University in Bangkok. She received her master's degree in health education from Chulalongkorn University, her second master's degree in community health nursing, and her DrPH from Mahidol University.

Julius J. Nam, PhD, JD, received his doctorate in religion from Andrews University where he wrote a dissertation on the relationship between Seventh-day Adventism and evangelical Protestantism in the United States. He has taught at Loma Linda University and Pacific Union College. He currently works for the US Department of Justice as an assistant United States attorney in Los Angeles, California.

Kwang-Hee Park, PhD, OMDLAC, received her doctoral degree in theology and personality from Claremont School of Theology and her doctorate in oriental medicine and acupuncture from South Baylo University in Orange County, California, where she worked as a researcher and patient counselor in the research department. She currently teaches both graduate courses in research, patient counseling, and psychology at South Baylo's department of Oriental medicine and herbology.

Manoj Shah, MD, is head of pediatrics gastroenterology division at Loma Linda University Medical Center and associate professor of pediatrics at Loma Linda University. He received his medical degree from Medical College, Baroda University in Gujarati, India and completed his residency at Cardinal Glennon Children's Hospital at St. Luke's Medical Center. He also served as vice president for the Federation of Gujarati Associations of North America, West Zone. He is the author of numerous peer-reviewed journal articles.

Siroj Sorajjakool, PhD, received his degree from Claremont School of Theology in the field of personality and theology and currently serves as professor of religion, psychology, and counseling at Loma Linda University. His research focus is on psychology among Asian religions.

Gerald Winslow, PhD, is the founding director of Loma Linda University's Institute for Health Policy and Leadership, and a professor of religion in the university's School of Religion. Previously, he served LLU as dean of the School of Religion, vice chancellor, and vice president for mission and culture. He received his undergraduate education at Walla Walla University and his master's degree at Andrews University. He earned his doctorate from Graduate Theological Union in Berkeley. He has also been a visiting scholar at Cambridge University, the University of Virginia, and the University of Tubingen. For over 40 years, he has specialized in teaching and writing about ethics, especially biomedical ethics. His current work focuses on the intersections of social and health policy. His books include *Triage and Justice* (University of California Press) and *Facing Limits* (edited with James Walters; Westview Press). His articles have appeared in academic journals such as *Western Journal of Medicine, Journal of Pediatrics, Hasting Center Report, Journal of Medicine and Philosophy,* and *General Dentistry.* He has presented seminars and lectures at universities and for professional groups throughout North America and in Australia, Europe, Russia, Africa, and Asia. He serves as the chairperson for Stakeholder Health's Advisory Council. He is also a member of the California Technology Assessment Forum, a public forum for the evaluation of new healthcare technologies. He has served as a consultant in biomedical ethics for major healthcare systems and for research conducted by pharmaceutical companies.

Preface

Teaching and publishing on the topic of world religions is not for the faint of heart. It takes courage and a bit of careless abandonment. Take, for instance, the idea that one can describe Hinduism in a single chapter – a religion that spans thousands of years, billions of adherents, and multiple continents, languages, and people groups. The same can be said for Islam, Christianity, Buddhism, Judaism, and so on.

Add to this the complexity of specific elements of each of these religions that have special relevance for healthcare. This effort is multifaceted. First, we seek to identify issues emerging from an authentic, lived-out, faith-based perspective on life and health. In other words, our aim is to convey information from within the religious context. Second, we must write and offer this work for the reader. Readers have specific needs – practical, educational needs that our authors must address. Third, when considering health beliefs and practices, it is difficult to make a clear distinction between faith and cultural practice.

Despite these challenges, we enthusiastically offer the text that follows. We are excited about it in part because we teach it and live it out in practice in the places we live and work. Most of the authors are, in fact, involved daily in teaching and/or practice that is focused on religion and healthcare. Faith-based healthcare institutions, both educational and service-oriented facilities, are hard pressed to thrive in the current context in North America. In a highly competitive and intensely difficult financial context, there remain people committed to offering healthcare from a faith-based perspective.

Regardless of the context from which you offer healthcare, providers must also be purposeful in this day and age to attend to matters of religion. The religious diversity that healthcare providers face in the lives of their patients is unprecedented in world history. North America is the most religiously diverse culture ever to appear and our healthcare providers must deal with this fact routinely.

We have assiduously approached this project from a non-partisan perspective. In other words, we are not offering this book for North American Christians to learn more about non-Christians they may face as clients and patients. Anyone who works in healthcare knows that as many, if not more, of the healthcare providers in North America are non-Christians. We do not need a book of the sort that looks toward the Other from a Christian or any one privileged perspective to see what they believe and who they are. The Hindu psychologist needs to know about Latter-day Saints as much as Catholic nurses need to know about Buddhists. The Muslim surgeon needs to know about Jehovah's Witness beliefs as much as the Sikh pharmacist needs to know about her Jewish patient. The Shi'a public health official needs to know more about the Sunni family who lives just down the street.

We find these inter-religious conversations to be incredibly energizing and useful. Useful to a society that celebrates its diversity. Useful to a community that purposefully seeks points of commonality while respecting points of difference. We hope that you will also.

There is very little storytelling in this volume, with the one notable exception of the chapter on American Indians. Although storytelling is integral to all religion, we made an exception in our format for the chapter on American Indians. The stories that will keep this volume alive in the minds of our readers, however, are those that you will share with your colleagues, friends, and families about what you have learned by reading; about what happened at work with this or that religious person or family or nurse or doctor. With our first edition, weeks prior to our deadline, we learned of a traditional Islamic practice of shaving the head of a newborn baby. As we finalized content for this edition, we are once again struck by a novel case of old believers from Russia here in America for three generations. Their death and burial rituals demanded they simply take their loved one's body from the ICU to their vehicle for transport home.

Preface to the second edition

We added two chapters to this second edition (Chapter 2: From conceptual to concrete and Chapter 6: Jainism). Besides these two chapters, Ernest J. Bursey made meaningful modifications to Chapter 1 and case studies on each religion have been added. In Chapter 2, Carr and Winslow offer a chapter that describes the interaction and methodological realities of ethics and religion/spirituality. Hospital-based clinical ethics in America (and abroad) have developed standards of case consultation the reader should know about. This need is based, in part, on the fact that ethics and religion are as intertwined and complex as is the question of culture and religion. And in the hospital context ethics have a direct bearing on how religion/ spirituality is lived out. This new chapter has a section focused on the ethics of caregiver–patient interaction with specific regard to religion and spirituality.

Additionally, Whitny Braun joins us with a chapter on Jainism. Dr. Braun writes from both personal experience and scholarly expertise in Jainism. Her work on Sallekhanā, a unique Jain ritual of fasting to death, recently took her to India to participate in the ongoing battle before the Supreme Court over the legality of the religious practice. Her research was featured in the appeal to overturn the court's decision to outright ban the practice and her testimony as an expert witness has been used by the lawyers arguing the case. Significantly high proportions of the Jain community are clinicians of allopathic medicine when compared to many of the other major religions, yet the group as a whole tends to avoid heroic measures in medicine and practice a careful ethic of not prescribing medication that may harm other life forms.

I would also like to express my appreciation to my colleagues who helped me identify and write the case studies included at the end of each chapter in this second edition. I wrote some of them, I co-authored some of them, and others authored some of them. Some of the authors I worked with were hesitant to identify themselves for fear that some involved parties might recognize elements of it. Although we masked personal identities, times, and locations out of respect for confidentiality (a subsidiary rule of the principle of respect for autonomy), a few authors did not want to be identified by name. Nonetheless, I owe them a note of gratitude and appreciation for their collaboration in this project.

While this is a collection of essays such that the individuality of each author is expressed in the essay, we offer it as a textbook that has a consistent chapter structure aimed at the reader's need for a useful reference on the various religious perspectives. These chapters illustrate the fact that the study of religion is an objective, scientific, and academic venture. We consider this academic exploration both essential and enriching. But for those who may read this text from a lived experience of faith, such an approach may be new and somewhat challenging.

A special thanks to the School of Religion for special funding to make this project a success; to Brianna Taylor for excellent work on abstracts for many chapters; to Brian Loui for researching demographic data, reformatting, completing abstracts, and adding final touches to the editorial process.

There is never a dull day in the offering of care to those in need. Religion is often a difficult, additional concern for already complex healthcare situations. But attending to patients' and families' religion is essential in our context. We commend you for your efforts and wish you well.

Mark F. Carr
Anchorage, July 2016

Foreword to the second edition

As *World Religions for Healthcare Professionals* advances to a second edition, I commend the editors who compiled this useful volume. Siroj Sorajjakool, Mark F. Carr, and Ernest J. Bursey have put together a work that has quickly shown its value to students in the classroom and professionals in the office.

In today's fast-changing society, books like this are essential for anyone who seeks to be knowledgeable of the world around. People are on the move, from East to West, immigrants or refugees. They bring with them their cultures and religions. Our neighbor, the clerk in the post office, the checker at the supermarket, the salesperson in the department store – we encounter Sikhs, Muslims, Buddhists, Hindus, and others of different faiths.

Inevitably, the doctor, dentist, or healthcare provider will be thrown into close encounters with clients from a variety of religious traditions. Sheer professionalism demands that the healthcare provider has a modicum of knowledge of the religious background of every patient in order to provide care with understanding and sensitivity. For many clients, even for those whose religion is the same as the professional, a visit to the office of the doctor, dentist, physical therapist, etc. in itself arouses apprehension. How much more is this the case when the client approaches with concerns that the professional may violate religious scruples or taboos?

This book meets an urgent and vital need. It is commendable, first, because those who write on each religious tradition actually practice that faith – they aren't arm-chair "experts." They know what matters, what sensibilities clients of that religion bring. Thus, while each writer lays out the basic tenets of the respective religion, each also gives specific, practical suggestions to enable the healthcare provider to avoid religious taboos.

While there are many works on world religion in the marketplace, this one stands apart because of its focus on health beliefs and practices. It targets, intentionally and specifically, the healthcare professional. A few other volumes attempt the same outcome, but they tend to be detailed in coverage and expensive to purchase. *World Religions for Healthcare Professionals* is concise, compact, and affordable.

I have assigned this book to students in my World Religions classes who are preparing for careers in dentistry, pharmacy, and other healthcare professions at Loma Linda University. They have found it useful. Now, as it is reprinted in a revised and expanded edition (a chapter on the Jain religion is added), it will be even more helpful.

William G. Johnsson, PhD
Loma Linda, California

1 Introduction

Ernest J. Bursey

Welcome to world religions from a healthcare perspective! The study of world religions offers you the opportunity to more adequately meet the needs of your patients and clients, because you will possess a more accurate knowledge of their religious beliefs and practices.

Extensive research supports the claim that patients who actively participate in a religion enjoy a longer life span and shorter stays in hospital than their counterparts. In a seminal, critical review, J. Levin (1994) concluded that the available published research at that time supported an association between religion and health, that the association is valid, and that it is probably causal. Subsequent research generally supports Levin's conclusion of a valid association between health and religion or spirituality. The *Handbook of Religion and Health*, a massive standard reference now in its second edition, estimates more than 2100 qualitative studies have been published, most indicating a positive correlation between religion and health (Koenig et al. 2012). A particularly important finding for our purposes is that the health benefits from religious affiliation are not restricted to one specific religion.

Evidence that the financial interests of a hospital are better served when the religious needs of patients are addressed while in the hospital has led to a growing use of spiritual assessment tools by both physicians and nurses, and the introduction of spirituality and medicine into the curricula of medical schools. In 1994, only 16 out of 126 medical schools offered courses in medicine and spirituality. By 2010, more than 90 percent of medical schools in America addressed spirituality and medicine in their curricula (Koenig et al. 2010).

The number of patients with religious affiliations other than Christianity has significantly increased because the general population of the United States has become more religiously diverse since 1965. That year, President Lyndon Johnson signed the Immigration and Nationality Act, which ended the national quota system that had discriminated against persons from Asia and the Middle East.

In the years since 1965, preferential access in immigration has been given to applicants with scientific and medical expertise needed in the

United States. For example, a study by Cornell University in 2002 disclosed that one in ten Muslim households in the United States includes a physician (Allied Media Corporation 2007). One positive benefit from the study of world religions could be a better understanding of the growing number of immigrant healthcare professionals who actively embrace a faith tradition other than Christianity. Nearly all of my graduate nursing students report working alongside nurses or physicians who openly hold to a faith other than their own and who believe their faith makes them better healthcare professionals.

Hopefully, as a result of reading this volume, you will become more aware of the religious minorities in your own community and perhaps more sensitive to the challenges they face in maintaining their religious practices and culture. The majority of legal immigrants, particularly from Central and South America, continue to be Christian since the largest percentage of immigrants to the United States are from Central and South America. But significant numbers of Hindus and Muslims, particularly from South Asia, have immigrated and become naturalized citizens. Mosques and temples sprout up in suburban American neighborhoods to meet the religious needs of the growing population of immigrants and their children. Funding for these projects is underwritten in part by affluent immigrant professionals, including those in healthcare and engineering. At the dedication of a new temple in Florida on June 15–19, 2005, a souvenir booklet itemized the names of donors; out of a total of 77 named devotees contributing $10,000 or more each, 42 were listed as "Dr.," with ten of these double listed as "Drs.," indicating both marriage partners held doctorates (Hindu Society of Central Florida 2005).

On a wider front, your knowledge about the religions of the world here in North America will give you one more window into understanding current events. Predictions of futurists a generation ago that organized religions would just wither away under the advance of secularism have turned out to be wrong. In the wider world, people are as prone as ever to identify with ancient religious traditions. Religious fundamentalism is alive and even growing within most of the major religions of the world, including Buddhism, Christianity, Hinduism, Islam, and Judaism. While religious difference is usually only one of several causes of armed conflicts, it often functions to give a justification for continuing conflicts between tribes or nations. The universally recognized Dalai Lama from Tibet has brought new luster to Buddhism while being castigated by the Chinese government for fomenting a separatist movement. Muslims around the world have been judged by the actions of the terrorists who flew the two airliners loaded with jet fuel into the Twin Towers on September 11, 2001. The declaration of a worldwide caliphate in 2014 by the Islamic State of Iraq and Syria (ISIS), a jihadist military group, and the response of disaffected young Muslims around the world to join the fighting has increased the fears that Islam is inherently bent on the overthrow of all governments, in spite of the denunciation against ISIS by virtually all Muslim scholars and religious leaders.

Personal benefits and challenges

We are more than healthcare professionals. We are, first of all, human beings who share with all human beings, including our patients, the mysteries of existence and the common experience of suffering and the certainty of death. As creatures with a bent to find meaning in our lives, we seek to cope with events that seem to defy any rational explanation. The medical explanation of an immediate cause for the death of a child falls short of explaining why we are living in a universe where this can happen. Religious people, like other humans, seek to find a conceptual framework that accounts for and even counters the apparent randomness of events. Religions attempt to answer the fundamental questions of why we have been born, the purpose of our existence, and what, if anything, lies beyond this life. It is true that when we begin to study another religion we are confronted with strange terms and even stranger practices that may give us the feeling that we are studying the beliefs of aliens quite different from ourselves. But at a deeper level, studying the religious beliefs of faiths other than your own may give you a sense of the deep bond you share with all other persons. Any medical care that fails to give homage to this common humanity dishonors the dignity of those it seeks to heal.

If you consider yourself an adherent of a particular religion, you may sense the inherent challenges, and even risks, in studying other religions. Students often discover they were misinformed about what a particular religion actually teaches, as a result of taking a course on world religions. Occasionally an introductory course in world religions leads to further study into a new religion and even the change of religious affiliation. A former student described being required as a child to attend her parents' church where she never felt at home with the ritual and loud preaching: "I often wanted to run out screaming." When she was an adult student in a world religions course, she chose to visit a Buddhist retreat center where she felt embraced within the serene setting and calmed by the instruction in meditation that reduced her inner stress. She called me from 2500 miles away to announce that she had found her true spiritual home. Her case is an exception. Much more often students challenged in a course in world religions decide to look more closely at their own religious tradition and acquire a more accurate knowledge of its basic beliefs. As any teacher of world religions can attest, most Americans, regardless of the religious tradition to which they belong, have a limited understanding of the resources of their own religious tradition. It has often been observed that by learning a second language a person develops a more acute understanding of one's native language. Likewise, a course in world religions often serves as a catalyst for a more mature grasp of a childhood faith.

While most healthcare professionals welcome the opportunity to better understand the religious perspectives of their clients and colleagues, not all are convinced, at least at the onset, of the need to spend time, effort, and expense to study the history and beliefs of various world religions. First, some are deeply convinced that their own religious faith is the only true one and that other religions teach dangerous ideas that can lead to the embrace of error, perhaps with eternal consequences. Typically persons holding this position also see it as their duty to share their beliefs with others, out of both a sense of responsibility and a concern for the welfare of others. Upon reflection, it becomes clear that any realistic attempt at sharing one's faith requires a sound knowledge of the beliefs and practices of the other. All persuasion begins on common ground. Given that the social decorum of healthcare professionals demands appropriate restrictions upon sharing one's faith, healthcare professionals living with a mandate to share their faith may live with an inner tension between the demands of their faith and their profession. Nonetheless, devout souls who await opportunities to speak of their faith are more likely to find receptive hearers if they are knowledgeable about the others' beliefs.

A second group that may be resistant to investing in the study of world religions are those who describe themselves as non-religious and who are aware of what they consider to be the harmful effects of religious dogmatism and superstition – wars, religious extremists, entrenched opposition to scientific knowledge and even to beneficial health practices. Concern for their patients' well-being may lead them to learn enough to avoid the pitfalls that would offend a devout patient. But a study of the worldviews and distinctive practices outside of the narrow healthcare arena seems irrelevant to the curriculum of a healthcare profession. It must be admitted that the non-religious or secular population is typically under-represented in courses on world religions. Perhaps you are part of that group. This marginalization masks the evidence that the secular or non-religious segment of American society, while still small, is growing in numbers and voice. Openly acknowledging the presence and the viewpoints of non-religious students is a vital step toward greater dialogue and engagement over the negative and positive influences of religion.

What is a world religion?

Ask ten people on the street for a definition of religion and you may get ten different answers, some focusing on the beliefs, some on practices or rituals. Even when scholars define religion, the results can be quite diverse, depending in part on whether a scholar is a sociologist or a psychologist, an anthropologist or a theologian. If the sociologist stresses the communal nature of religious practice and the social construction of religious beliefs, the psychologist may address religion within the individual's search for autonomy and personhood. The anthropologist stands outside the circle of religious belief in describing myth and ritual within a specific cultural context, while the theologian presumes the possibility of communication with a supernatural reality. For the purposes of this book, rather than hammering out a definition of religion, our efforts can be better spent in identifying and comparing the features that are common to different religions and then to recognize the functions that religions and religious beliefs have.

Where do I come from? Why am I here? What happens after death? Religion can be understood as a response to these questions of human origin, purpose, and destination, especially in the light of the certainty of death and the uncertainties of life. The mystery of our own existence and the realization that we are transient creatures attracts many to religions that claim access to the unseen beyond the senses. Each day we are immersed in a stream of events that arrive without warning. Religions typically offer the believer some sort of coherent framework of meaning to interpret these apparently random events. Religions also issue directives on how we might impose a semblance of order in our daily lives through the observance of times of worship, prayer, reading of sacred texts, and meditation.

The focus of this volume is the so-called "world religions," although Native American religions and new religious movements are included. Humans are universally religious. Yet not every religion can be called a world religion. When academics refer to world religions, the list typically includes Hinduism, Buddhism, Islam, Judaism, Taoism, Confucianism, and Christianity. Other religions occasionally included are Sikhism, Jainism, Zoroastrianism, and the Baha'i. Shinto, the national religion of Japan, and nature religions such as Wicca may be included as well. In addition to being widespread, the so-called "world religions" typically possess scriptures or religious texts that serve to anchor religious beliefs and written collections of authoritative teachings that can be transmitted from one generation to the next. Jews revere the Tanakh and study the rulings of rabbis found in the Mishnah and Talmud. Muslims consider the Qur'an to contain the very words of Allah and draw on the preserved rulings of legal scholars familiar with the collections of sayings about and by Muhammad. But humans have been religious long before they learned to transmit knowledge through the medium of writing. Throughout the world and on every inhabited continent, indigenous peoples have feared unseen spiritual forces and sought to control them or seek their favor, often by elaborate ritual and the observance of taboos.

Religion and culture

This textbook focuses on religions and on the religious beliefs and practices that are characteristic of religions, not on culture and cultural practices. But religion is a part of culture. Culture includes the totality of the customs and practices of a distinct group of people. So separating what is religious from what is simply cultural is not an easy matter. It might seem that the beliefs and rituals of a world religion like Buddhism or Islam or Christianity ought to be the same anywhere in the world. Yet the way a religion is actually practiced may vary considerably from culture to culture, and age to age. Labels like "fundamentalist," "conservative," "progressive," and "liberal" are used to describe the variations within a religion and suggest that the individual variations in religious practices may not be isolated but part of a larger collection of specific practices and beliefs considered as "core" for groups within a given religion.

Deciding what belongs under the umbrella of religion can be complicated and even confusing. Persons living in one country may include rituals or customs as part of their religious obligations that persons belonging to the same religion but living in a different country consider optional or even refuse to practice. For instance, the practice of female genital mutilation or female circumcision is widely practiced in Egypt. According to a recent study, 92 percent of Egyptian women have undergone some form of female circumcision (Ministry of Health and Population et al. 2015: 185). The Egyptian government made the procedure illegal in 2008. Yet the practice persists. A frequently cited reason is the belief that good Muslim women undergo the operation. In contrast to the societal encouragement in Egypt, the conservative Muslim society of nearby Saudi Arabia looks down upon the practice as against the principles of Islam. Saudi Arabia has legally forbidden the procedure as well.

Who then decides whether a belief or practice is to be truly considered a religious obligation or simply a traditional cultural practice? In some religions, a recognized religious authority may make the decision about what is core and non-negotiable. Roman Catholics generally consider the decisions of popes, past and present, to define what they are to believe and practice. In some religions, there may be no comparable, universally recognized figure or authoritative group. More than 50 percent of Egyptian women still consider female circumcision to be a religious requirement (Ministry of Health and Population et al. 2015: 185). High-ranking religious leaders claiming otherwise are dismissed because they are government funded.

The impact of American culture on transplanted faith traditions is often profound. Immigrants who come to the United States from a country where their religion was sponsored by the government discover on arriving that if they want to retain their religious faith they must take more personal initiative in the practice of their religion than they had taken in their country of origin. The openness and even secularization of American culture can have a double-edge effect on religious minorities – on the one hand, leading to a deepening personal understanding of one's faith, but on the other hand, raising legitimate concerns about the religious commitments of the second and third generation. I recall a Muslim businesswoman from Tanzania telling the students in my classroom that she knew more about her faith and why she was a Muslim than her relatives who remained in Tanzania, where their religion was taken for granted and supported by loudspeakers announcing the times of prayer.

Scholars of religions in America note that transported religions, including even the major world religions, tend to morph into more distinctly American forms. The openness of American culture makes isolation difficult. A continual infusion of new immigrants ensures the retention of traditional practices and views. But over time, something uniquely American or Westernized begins to emerge. Factors that drive this on-going process include the expectation of American women to fully participate and even lead out in religious functions, the constitutional freedom to openly discuss and debate religious matters, the recognized absolute right of personal choice in matters of faith, and the acceptance of inter-faith marriages. Debates over the physical presence of women in public worship continue to percolate in traditional Muslim and Orthodox Jewish communities.

The desire of immigrants to lessen prejudice by blending into the cultural landscape and to demonstrate loyalty to an adopted country leads to changes in the practice of their religion. R. H. Seager observes an indigenous American Buddhism in the making, though the process is far from completed (Seager 2002: 118). Japanese farmers immigrated to America in the 1800s, bringing their Shin Buddhist religion with them. Over time, temples were built that outwardly imitated the appearance of Protestant churches, unlike the traditional architecture of Shin Buddhist temples in Japan. Pews replaced mats. Western musical instruments, hymns, and even choirs were incorporated into the religious services. After the Japanese attack on Pearl Harbor in 1941 and President Roosevelt's executive order to round up citizens of Japanese descent, the name, Buddhist Mission of North America, was changed to Buddhist Churches of America.

Other transplanted religions face similar developments. Santeria, a New World version of the African Yoruba religion, was twice transplanted, first as early as the sixteenth century by slaves to Cuba where they found common ground between African gods and Catholic saints and managed to continue their devotion to the orishas disguised as saints. The religion was transported a second time by exiles fleeing to the United States during Fidel Castro's revolution. Most of the estimated adherents in the States are now light-skinned, college educated, and middle class. Of interest to healthcare professionals is the vast healing lore involving herbalists and spiritualist mediums. Coming out from the shadows of secrecy in the more permissive and pluralistic American environment, the first Santeria church was established in Hialeah, Florida in 1974. The religion appears to be growing in numbers; estimates of devotees range from half a million upwards. Meanwhile, the previously required animal sacrifices are decreasing and drumming is avoided out of respect for neighbors (De La Torre 2004: 205–23).

On the other hand, the growing impact of religious beliefs and practices from immigrant religions is equally noteworthy, especially in healthcare. Payment for Chinese acupuncture treatment is widely, if not universally, accepted by insurance plans. Mindfulness, part of the Eightfold Path of Buddhism, is securely embedded in hospitals and university research centers as a legitimate therapy for stress and stress-related illness. The impetus to introduce Buddhist mindfulness practice into secular American healthcare using non-religious vocabulary is credited to Jon Kabat-Zinn, former Professor of Medicine at the University of Massachusetts. Faith-based hospitals in the Christian tradition have resisted what has been described as "stealth Buddhism" (Brown 2014). Yoga as a way to improve one's health is now as American as apple pie, notwithstanding protests from Hindu purists and some religious voices in the Christian and Islamic traditions.

Religion, ethics, and transformation

While religions have traditionally focused on how we ought to relate to the divine, all the major religions of the world also promote moral codes of conduct about how we ought to relate to each other. Whether you look in the Jewish Tanakh, the Christian New Testament, the Buddhist Dhammapada, the Hindu Bhagavad Gita, or the Muslim Qur'an, these codes of conduct are actually quite similar in forbidding murder, adultery, stealing, lying, disrespect of parents and elders, etc. The Golden Rule attributed to Jesus in the New Testament, "Do to others what you would want them to do to you," can be paralleled by the words of Muhammad, Buddha, and other religious teachers. Some Americans fear that basic moral standards will be undermined by the growing number of the population that embrace non-Christian religions. Such fears are groundless. Religions of the world generally place a high value on honesty, unselfishness, marital faithfulness, and the responsibility to preserve human life. Religious persons of every stripe tend to oppose abortion or the practice of active euthanasia at higher rates than more secular persons.

All the major religions of the world also address the contradictions of human behavior in that humans typically live below the standards of their own moral codes, with some falling far short of basic human decency. These lapses require both an explanation and an antidote. The religions of the world tend to diverge from one another in their diagnosis of the cause for that gap between acceptable standards and actual moral conduct. It is not surprising that differing etiologies to account for moral failure lead to divergent prescriptions or strategies for closing the moral gap. Hindus and Buddhists expect reincarnation or rebirth to deal with negative karma accumulated from wrong-doing in previous lives. Muslims practice the regimen of submissive prayer five times daily as an aid to keeping their mind on the straight path of righteousness. Christians hold to the benefits from a crucified Savior to counter the consequences of a fatally flawed human nature.

A note about the "nones"

The percentage of Americans claiming no religious affiliation rose dramatically from 16 percent to 23 percent in the seven years from 2007 to 2014. A closer look reveals important differences among these "nones." But every category shows a trend away from organized religion (Lipka 2016). This trend appears to follow the pattern of European secularization. Some find no interest or value in the discussion or practice of religion. In 2014, one in ten Americans fell into this simply secular category of no interest. If all persons adopted this position, books and courses about world religions would cease, except for the study of religion as a cultural artifact of the past. Age comparisons are even more alarming to those who see religious belief as a bulwark of morality. While two-thirds of those born before 1946 claim religion to be important in their lives, the number for those born between 1981 and 1996 drops to only four out of ten (Gjelten 2015). Efforts to understand and counter these trends are evident in every faith tradition.

Factors toward the marginalization of religion and the drop in religious affiliation include a sense that science conveys truth while religion may peddle tradition; the lack of confidence in the relevance of religious organizations; the publicized moral corruption of religious leaders; and, in the case of Christianity and Islam, a rejection of an angry or vengeful God. The plurality of religions can create a disbelief that any of them can claim to provide the exclusive avenue to the Divine.

Seven percent of the population are not affiliated with a specific religion but believe a religious or spiritual perspective to be important. These are typically categorized as "spiritual but not religious" (SBNR). Often they "have rejected a God stereotyped as a judgment overseer and instead have substituted the idea of a sacred force which is impersonal and benevolent" (Mercadante 2014: 230). A self-declared former SBNR, Mercadante notes that many will in time move from the category of "none" to affiliate with a religion. The search for a coherent meaning to human existence and for religious practices to counteract a self-centered spiritual experience and for the strength that comes from belonging can lead them to a religious community. Ideally, that community is able to portray a loving God and offer a counter view to the values of a market-driven culture.

Another 3 percent polled considered themselves atheists, double the percentage in 2007; while self-identified agnostics also almost doubled at 4 percent in 2014. Two out of three atheists are males, with a median age of 34, compared with a median age of 46 for the general public. Deep suspicion of atheists shows up, with 51 percent of Americans viewing atheism as a personal deterrent when voting for the President, down from

63 percent in 2007. Recently the strident calls of prominent atheists like Richard Dawkins and Christopher Hitchens to eliminate religious belief and abolish religious privileges have found a widespread audience. But other atheists recognize the social value of religion and seek to establish corresponding non-theistic or humanist communities that can work with religious organizations in bettering human life (Stedman 2013, cited in Krattenmaker 2016).

Religion and healthcare

One of the distinctive features of this textbook on world religions is the focus on healthcare. Historically, virtually all religions have been concerned with illness and the maintenance of health. Some offer explanations for the presence of sickness and death. Some paradigms for treating illness are theoretically tied to particular religions. Ayurveda, a form of medical care widely practiced in India and to some extent in North America as an alternative to Western medicine, is closely associated with Hinduism. Traditional Chinese medicine, including acupuncture and moxibustion, has theoretical roots in Taoist thought. On the other hand, the missionary religions of Buddhism, Christianity, and Islam have not been so closely tied to a particular medical paradigm, but their followers have accommodated to a variety of medical practices.

For thousands of years, religion has been involved in bringing physical and mental healing. Illness has been widely considered as caused by negative or even hostile spiritual forces that need to be appeased or even banished to restore health. Jesus, the founder of Christianity, healed the sick, often by means of exorcism, alongside his preaching. His enemies attributed his particular effectiveness as an exorcist to an alleged alliance with Satan. A key factor in the spread of Christianity was the perceived effectiveness of Christian missionaries in banishing evil spirits in the name of Jesus. Yet today physicians in the west who call themselves Christians typically do not include demonic possession as a diagnosis. Florida Hospital, a faith-based Christian hospital with the motto "Extending the healing ministry of Christ," does not have a department of exorcism but follows the protocols of Western biomedical healthcare. Yet many devout believers continue to put their confidence in prayers and rituals to address what they consider to be the spiritual causes of their illness. Whether or not you hold such views, you will need to become aware of the differing understandings of illness in order to more skillfully assist your patients in their recovery.

The rapid growth of medical knowledge has raised profound challenges to the ethical norms of all the world religions. Religious leaders have struggled to keep up in providing the faithful with guidance regarding life-creating, life-extending, and life-denying technologies that were previously unimaginable but now are readily available. Rather than automatically embracing the latest life-enhancing miracle or simply denouncing the new outright, they have more often turned to their scriptures, the ancient texts held to contain the essential wisdom, in order to provide a rationale for embracing or denying each medical advance. Shall sperm donors be denounced as adulterers? Does *in vitro* fertilization blur the distinction between the Creator and the human creature? Is the circulation of blood through external cleansing equipment during surgery a violation of the Bible's prohibition against ingesting blood?

If God is the source of human life, under what circumstances then, if any, may a pregnancy be terminated? Muslim and Catholic theologians differ on when an embryo receives a soul or is deemed a person, and consequently they issue different rulings regarding the use of drugs that impede implantation of the embryo in the lining of the uterus.

When is the removal of artificial life support justified? Religions typically place a high value on human life and stand almost united against active euthanasia or physician-assisted suicide. Yet limits to the utilization of life-extending technology have to be drawn somewhere. In most religions, the authority of a religious leader will be recognized by only a portion of the faithful and so conflicting views may be offered as options. The Orthodox Jewish belief that the soul of a person gradually withdraws from the body and may remain with the body even when higher brain function appears to cease can put end-of-life decisions on a collision course between medical personnel and the dying person's family. These conflicts make graphic headlines in newspapers eager to boost reader interest: "Catholic godson of woman on life support fights to get proxy back" (Saul 2014) and "Hasidic boy in legal fight over life support buried" (Furse 2008). Chayim Aruchim, a program of the ultra-conservative Agudath Israel of America, appeals to Jews to seek the guidance of a rabbi trained in Jewish law or halakha when navigating end-of-life issues. For a comprehensive guide to the range of Orthodox halakha reasoning, see Shabtai (2012). Less conservative Jews in the Reformed and Conservative branches of Judaism are more likely to end life support when no brain activity can be detected and the beating heart is dependent on a mechanical ventilator.

The importance of preserving the body intact for a future resurrection of the deceased has often stood in the way of Muslim, Jewish, and Catholic families granting permission for medical autopsy for potentially valuable medical knowledge. Autopsy itself has seemed to some to be like the desecrating of the fallen warrior on the field of battle, forbidden by the sacred text of the Qur'an. Yet when organ transplantation offered the gift of life to persons dying from organ failure, theologians and religious leaders reconsidered long-held positions and took up the questions of when organs could be harvested, who should receive them, etc. When the faithful accept the gift of an organ for the sake of preserving their own lives, fairness calls for reciprocity by allowing them to offer that gift to another person.

A recommendation to enhance your learning

This text was carefully prepared by knowledgeable experts to offer you a reliable overview of the several recognized world religions. Yet I recommend that you supplement a careful reading of this text with face-to-face conversations with persons from other religious traditions who are active in the practice of their own religion. I know of no other experience to better awaken your awareness of what you have been reading.

Reading a chapter in this book about a religion other than your own will serve to introduce you to that tradition. It would require years of careful study and experience for a Christian, for instance, to know the vast range of views and practices that are held among so-called Hindus. Should you interview a person from another religious tradition, you may discover that this person holds views about their religion that differ somewhat from what is found in the chapter on that religion in this textbook. On the other hand, if you read the chapter carefully in advance of the interview, you may discover that you know specific information about that religion or its history that the person you interview did not know about their own religion! Most importantly, you will learn not so much about the religion's beliefs and history but how another person actually practices the religion they love. That is a treasure worth seeking.

Conclusion

As you study each of the religions, picture in your mind four concentric circles. In the outer and largest circle, you will find the basic information about a world religion's belief system and resources, as well as how it is practiced with some variations around the world.

Then picture inside that larger circle a smaller circle to represent how that religion is practiced here in the United States where religious freedom is practiced but where Christianity is the dominant religion. The inevitable impact of American culture produces accommodations and innovations in each incoming religion. Conversely, incoming religions enrich American culture. In this textbook, you will find some attention to this circle of cultural immersion. Likely you will find further evidence of accommodation if you take up the suggestion of interviewing a person from another religious tradition.

Now envision a still smaller circle to represent American healthcare. Here the religious beliefs and practices of patients and healthcare practitioners interact with one another. When faced with medical issues, patients from every religious tradition draw from their own spiritual wells. A significant part of every chapter will be spent considering that inner circle of the intersection of healthcare and religion.

Finally, you can imagine an even smaller circle to represent your own religious traditions, practices, and beliefs. In this course on the major religions of the world, you will have the opportunity to reflect on your own religious traditions, practices, and beliefs, should you wish to do so. I hope that you will take advantage of this opportunity.

Studying and working in the field of healthcare prompts one to see that we are living in a time of change. Buddhist, Christian, Hindu, and Muslim healthcare professionals are caring for patients of all faiths and denominations in American hospitals and clinics. Not everywhere yet. But the tides of change continue to spread. Will we learn how to work together with our cultural and religious differences? Will we be able to hold on to our old exclusionary ideas of "us" and "them?" Or will we make larger inclusive circles of commitment and care that respect and even value this religious diversity? Your study of world religions from a healthcare perspective will give you the confidence you need to join the larger circle.

Bibliography

Allied Media Corporation (2007) "American Muslims." Available online at: www.allied-media.com/AM (accessed December 8, 2008).

Brown, C. G. (2014) "Mindfulness: Stealth Buddhism for mainstreaming meditation?" *The Huffington Post*, December 2, 2014, updated February 1, 2015. Available online at: www.huffingtonpost.com/candy-gunther-brown-phd/mindfulness-stealth-buddh_b_6243036.html (accessed June 29, 2016).

Chayim Aruchim. Website of the Chayim Aruchim, Center for Culturally Sensitive End-of-Life Advocacy and Counseling. Available online at: www.chayima-ruchim.com/Pages/aboutUs (accessed June 15, 2016).

De La Torre, M. (2004) *Santeria: Beliefs and Rituals of a Growing Religion in America*, Grand Rapids, MI: Wm. B. Eerdmans.

Furse, J. H. (2008) "Hasidic boy in legal fight over life support buried," *New York Daily News*, November 17, 2008. Available online at: www.nydailynews.com/ny_local/brooklyn/2008/11/16/2008-11-16_hasidic_boy_in_legal_fight_over_life_sup.html (accessed June 29, 2016).

Gjelten, T. (2015) "Poll finds Americans, especially millennials, moving away from religion," *The Two Way: Breaking News from NPR*, November 3, 2015. Available online at: www.npr.org/sections/thetwo-way/2015/11/03/454063182/poll-finds-americans-especially-millennials-moving-away-from-religion (accessed June 29, 2016).

Hindu Society of Central Florida (2005) *MahaKumbabhishekam and Prathistapanam Celebrations, June 15–19, 2005, Souvenir and Directory*, Casselberry, FL: Hindu Society of Central Florida. Current lists of trustees and patrons are available at: www.hindutempleorlando.org.

Koenig, H. G., Hooten, E. G., and Lindsay-Calkins, E. (2010) "Spirituality in medical school curricula: Findings from a national survey," *International Journal of Psychiatry in Medicine*, vol. 40, no. 4: 391–8.

Koenig H. G., King, D. E., and Carson, V. B. (2012) *Handbook of Religion and Health*, 2nd edn, New York, NY: Oxford University Press.

Krattenmaker, T. (2016) "The 'nones' are becoming somethings," *Reflections Yale Divinity School*, Spring, 2016: 44–5. Available online at: http://reflections.yale.

edu/article/all-together-now-pluralism-and-faith/nones-are-becoming-somethings (accessed June 29, 2016).

Levin, J. (1994) "Religion and health: Is there an association, is it valid, and is it causal?," *Social Science and Medicine*, vol. 38, no. 11: 1475–82.

Lipka, M. (2016) "Ten facts about atheists," *Pew Research Center*, June 1, 2016. Available online at: www.pewresearch.org/fact-tank/2016/06/01/10-facts-about-atheists/ (accessed June 2, 2016).

Mercadante, L. A. (2014) *Belief Without Borders: Inside the Minds of the Spiritual but not Religious*, New York, NY: Oxford University Press.

Ministry of Health and Population, El-Zanaty and Associates, and ICF International (2015) *Egypt Demographic and Health Survey 2014*, Cairo, Egypt and Rockville, Maryland, USA: Ministry of Health and Population and ICF International. Available online at: http://dhsprogram.com/pubs/pdf/FR302/FR302.pdf (accessed June 29, 2016).

Saul, J. (2014) "Catholic godson of woman on life support fights to get proxy back," *New York Post*, March 20, 2014. Available online at http://nypost.com/2014/03/20/catholic-godson-of-woman-on-life-support-fights-to-get-proxy-back/ (accessed June 29, 2016).

Seager, R. H. (2002) "American Buddhism in the making," in Prebish, C. S. and Baumann, M. (eds) *Westward Dharma: Buddhism beyond Asia*, Berkeley, CA: University of California Press.

Shabtai, D. (2012) *Defining the Moment: Understanding Brain Death in Halakah*, New York, NY: Shoresh Press.

Stedman, C. (2013) *How an Atheist Found Common Ground with the Religious*, Boston, MA: Beacon Press.

2 From conceptual to concrete

Mark F. Carr and Gerald R. Winslow

Some people are more inclined to broad, theoretical views of life while others are more concerned with the practical matters and particular details of everyday life (Jonsen 1991: 14–16). Both patterns of thought are essential in religion and healthcare. The methods of decision making and patient care detailed below take this into account. Nationally and internationally, these two modes of thought are associated with two methods of clinical decision making in healthcare. Principles-based reasoning, or what has come to be called principlism, as well as case-based reasoning, or casuistry, are both highly influential in the field of ethics and morality in healthcare decision making.

Principles-based patient care

There are four principles that are widely accepted as essential for morally appropriate patient care. *Respect for autonomy, beneficence, nonmaleficence*, and *justice* have emerged from centuries of religious, social, and cultural attention to religion and morality. The institutions of our civilization have been significantly shaped by shared conceptions and applications of these four principles. Though there is debate about exactly how many principles suffice to capture the essence of this common morality, with some arguing for as many as seven, the most influential advocates of principlism assert that these four are sufficient (Beauchamp and Childress 2013: 2–13).

Before proceeding to a discussion of how the principles may be applied in the clinical setting, it will be helpful to provide a brief definition for each of the four:

- *Respect for autonomy*: respecting the choices of the patient. In recent decades, especially starting in the 1970s with the promulgation of the "Patients' Bill of Rights," much greater emphasis was placed on the ethical importance of honoring the patient's expressed values and decisions.
- *Beneficence*: ensuring the patient receives significant benefit from healthcare interventions. Patients generally trust their professional

caregivers to give priority to the good of the patient over other potentially competing concerns. Seeking the patient's good is what the healthcare professions, in their codes of ethics, all profess.

- *Nonmaleficence*: guarding against harming the patient. One of the most time-honored commitments of healthcare professionals is captured in an oft-repeated Latin expression – *primum non nocere* – which means "first of all, do not harm."
- *Justice*: treating patients equitably, without unfair discrimination. The essence of this principle is a commitment to human equality with differences in treatment based on morally relevant considerations.

According to the most prevalent view of principlism, the four principles are not hierarchical; they are not to be considered in rank order since one is no more or less important than the others. Rather, they move in and out of relevance in any given case as details of the case are discovered and capture our attention. Based upon the case details, typically one of the principles will supersede the others. The careful work of figuring out which of the principles should take priority in any particular case is the responsibility of caregivers and the people for whom they are caring. Let us illustrate:

A two-car accident involving a 24-year-old male alone in his vehicle and a family of five in a minivan brings out the paramedics. Upon arrival at the scene the family is found to have only minor injuries, but the young man has passed out from shock primarily due to a compound fracture of his left femur. He has lost a lot of blood. Paramedics do their best to revive him, and upon further assessment they believe that he probably also sustained a number of internal injuries. They rush him to the emergency room (ER) while trying to contact his family.

As principles-based reasoning goes, thus far in the case the paramedics have correctly responded under the principle of beneficence; they clearly are doing good for the patient, trying to keep him alive. Doing good for persons in distress is an immediate, intuitive, and also learned response for both lay and professional people in our society. In the ER, these beneficent responses are well established. Thus, it would seem rather odd, given this brief case description, for anyone in the emergency setting to appeal to other principles, such as justice. Nor is anyone likely to wonder if we are actually harming this young man (nonmaleficence). Since he is unconscious, it would also be nonsensical to ask him for his informed consent under the principle of respect for autonomy.

Imagine, however, that the details of the case shift rather quickly. Within the next couple of hours, the man's wife and extended family arrive at the ER with his advance healthcare directive in hand. The directive clearly indicates that he does not want any blood products in the event of a serious accident or critical illness. This is because he is a Jehovah's Witness and he holds religious convictions that forbid the use of blood products for medical care.

Within the next hour of treatment in the ER, the young man's condition continues to decline. While the fracture and associated bleeding are managed, the internal bleeding continues. His wife and family refuse to give consent for surgery, again citing the use of blood products. After considerable argument between the ER physicians and the family (the patient was still unconscious), the physicians and hospital administrators decide to seek a court order to allow them to take the young man to surgery and use the full measure of blood products and methods at their disposal. Thus, the hospital risk management team takes a request to the judge on call in the hope of getting an injunction that will allow them to use blood products. The judge rules in favor of the patient's family, thus effectively giving priority to respect for the patient's autonomy as expressed through his advance directive.

Principles-based reasoning is again at work here. One of the important reasons for an advance healthcare directive is to honor the personal choices of patients. Of course, these personal choices are routinely, deeply influenced by our religion and spirituality. Thus, respect for autonomy comes to the fore as an important principle to consider in this specific case at this specific time. In light of the patient's religious desire to avoid the use of blood, the principle of beneficence is now in conflict with the principle of respect for autonomy. Additionally, if the ER team were to simply override the family's desire to honor his advance directive, one could argue that they would actually be harming the patient, thereby breaking the principle of nonmaleficence (avoiding harm) in the process.

While the family members are clear that they do not want their loved one to die, they do not want to override his clearly expressed religious convictions. And with frustrated reluctance, the ER team accepts the judge's decision to honor the young man's advance directive. There will be no surgery without the family's consent, and the ER must not use any blood products in caring for the young man. Despite their best efforts, the young man dies within the hour following the judge's decision.

The process of specifying and balancing the four principles is a crucial skill in the principles-based method of caring for patients (Beauchamp and Childress 2013: 17–24). Critical thinking skills and self-reflective practices are essential tools for any clinician seeking to care appropriately for patients. It is part of clinicians' professional responsibility to evaluate the relevance of each of the principles and determine which of them will take priority over the others at any given point in the case.

For nearly four decades, through several editions of *Principles of Biomedical Ethics*, the four principles just mentioned have continued to be extensively influential. Meanwhile, international attention to a principles-based approach has also generated guidance worth noting. For example, in 1998 the "Final Report to the European Commission on the Project, Basic Ethical Principles in Bioethics and Biolaw, 1995–1998" was published. Occasionally referred to as the *Barcelona Declaration*, the document details a different set of four principles: *autonomy, dignity, integrity*, and *vulnerability*. Seven years later, the United Nations (UNESCO division) offered the "Universal Declaration of Bioethics and Human Rights." Using a far more expansive list of 15 principles, this document now serves the international community on matters of religion and ethics in clinical medicine. Of particular usefulness to our concern for religion and healthcare, Articles 8, 11, and 12 are noteworthy. Article 8, "Respect for human vulnerability and personal integrity," acknowledges patients' vulnerability but also includes personal integrity. Below, we will detail further how these two concerns are closely linked in attending to patients' religious and spiritual needs and resources. Article 11, "Non-discrimination and non-stigmatization," and Article 12, "Respect for cultural diversity and pluralism," further express a commitment to care for patients in ways that are fully respectful of their personhood, including their religious identity, or lack thereof.

Closely associated with principlism is another prominent method of attending to religion and morality, referred to as "casuistry" or the "four-box" method. For ease of memory, we refer to it as "case-based" as it is compared and contrasted to the principles-based approach.

Case-based patient care

The proponents of the case-based approach, Albert Jonsen, Mark Siegler, and William Winslade, offered their model in stark contrast and opposition to the principles-based model (Jonsen et al. 2015). Over time, however, both camps have conceded some points, and both have incorporated some of the more persuasive elements of the others' arguments. For the case-based group, the method consists of attending to four crucial details of the actual case; they want to know (1) the medical conditions, (2) the patient's preferences, (3) the patient's quality of life, and (4) contextual features of the patient's case. The authors have depicted these four considerations in a four-quadrant table, with medical conditions and patient's preferences in the upper two quadrants, and quality of life and contextual features in the lower two quadrants. Early on, the authors expressed the belief that more than 90 percent of all cases could be resolved within the medical conditions quadrant, followed by sequential progression through the other three quadrants, as described above. Over time, however, the proponents have modulated this sequential, four-box approach in favor of giving more holistic attention to the entirety of the quadrants. At the back of their book, they have even provided a removable card-stock page in order to facilitate having the four quadrants, with their accompanying questions, readily available.

Given the pragmatic and often fast-paced context of inpatient care, this case-based approach has gained popularity with medical doctors when treating complex cases, including those in which the patient's religion represents a significant consideration. The hefty, in-depth volume of the *Principles of Biomedical Ethics* makes it the preference of professors and philosophers of medical humanities and ethics. While both publications express respect for religious convictions and diversity, neither of them gives extensive attention to religion and spirituality. Beauchamp and Childress (2013) argue that religion and spirituality are so pervasive throughout the entirety of our common morality that treating them as standalone topics would be disingenuous. Jonsen, Siegler, and Winslade, on the other hand, simply embed religion in their fourth box, "Contextual Features," with the following question: "Are there religious factors that might influence clinical decisions?" (Jonsen et al. 2015).

When resolving difficult clinical cases, including those with significant religious factors, healthcare professionals will be well-served by either method described above, or by some combination of methods in what some refer to as "reflective equilibrium" (Rawls 1971: 20). This expression, coined by philosopher John Rawls, points out the reality that our reasoned judgments, guided by established principles, are routinely adjusted by the specific details of any given case (Beauchamp and Childress 2013: 404–410). In similar fashion, our understanding of principles matures over time as we gain experience in their application to specific cases. In essence, this argument says that justification for a normative position taken in response to a religious or ethical quandary is found in the reasoning of both principles-based and case-based methods. The two are better understood as complementary rather than as competitors.

The need for more

There are three additional approaches to clinical ethics that need careful consideration if we are to create a comprehensive and ethically effective response to religious and spiritual concerns in the clinical setting. We address these under the rubrics of *narrative ethics*, *virtue ethics*, and *care ethics*. The additional insights and practical guidance from these approaches have considerable value in the clinical care of patients.

Narrative ethics

Have you ever asked someone a clear and pointed question only to have her or him respond by telling a story? A former student referred to being angry at her father when she was young because every time she asked him a hard question, he would sit back and tell her a story. She never really understood, until she heard the description of narrative faith and ethics. This approach features the central importance of stories – stories that form the essence of our religion, ethics, and spirituality. These are not limited to an individual's own personal stories, but they may also be the stories of one's family, community, church, school, state, nation, and so forth. Human beings are so deeply embedded in such stories that it would be impossible to resolve religious and moral dilemmas in ways that do not attend to the stories that shape the involved person's understanding of the context.

People hear, interpret, and repeat meaningful stories every day. Among the most powerful of these are the religious stories that thoroughly shape the lives of billions of people. Without the story of Siddhartha, what would Buddhism be? Without Muhammad, how would we understand the story of Islam? Christianity without Jesus is unthinkable. And lest anyone think this approach works only for religion, we might ask what of the United States of America, without George Washington? Or the Republic of South Africa without Nelson Mandela?

Hilde Lindemann Nelson identifies at least five things we do with stories that may profoundly affect how we live our lives: (1) *reading* stories, (2) *telling* stories, (3) *comparing* stories, (4) *analyzing* stories, and (5) *invoking* stories. All five of these, according to the author, are part of the process of making sense of life (Nelson 1997: x–xii). In the realm of health and illness, it is often the case that the power of religious and spiritual stories is dramatically enhanced. It is hard to overstate the thoroughgoing nature of this approach to life and religion. One narrative theorist in medical contexts, Kathryn Montgomery Hunter, insists that "narrative is the primary way of organizing and communicating" what it means to be human in our world. At the "heart of human knowing" lies an "interpretive process integral to shaping and understanding" our lives through story (Hunter 2004). Indeed, from this perspective, religion is unintelligible without thoroughgoing engagement in telling stories.

Young people may often be bored or annoyed with having to sit through the stories their parents or grandparents tell, some of which may be told over and over again. Yet, as those same young people themselves grow older, they often find themselves remembering and perhaps even recounting the same stories. Whether or not it is realized, the subconscious effects of stories shape the way we live and function in the world.

Often the intention of telling religious stories is to lead the hearers (or readers) to accept practical lessons. "Now boys and girls, the moral of the story is..." is the oft-used transition away from the details of the story itself to the lessons that children are supposed to learn from the story. Narrative religionists are prone to point out that the stories, in and of themselves, are strong enough to convey the lessons. There is no need to moralize at the end of the story. A crucial task for responsible humans, who share a concern for enhancing the spiritual and religious lives of their community, is simply to tell the stories well (Hauerwas and Jones 1989: 158–190).

In clinical care, much may be learned about patients by listening attentively to their stories. In particular, when patients reach the end of their lives, families often need to retell the stories that have been important to them through the years. As much as possible, caregivers may help provide time for this process. Additionally, those caring for dying patients and their family members can use stories to help them understand and process what is going on in their dying process.

Attending to patients' life stories highlights *respect for autonomy*. Listening to family stories about their religion and the proper practice of it near the end of life brings ongoing meaning in family life. One of the case studies used in this text dramatically highlighted this reality for palliative care nurse practitioner Marianne Johnston-Petty. Thinking she understood how a 34-year-old Christian man would go about making decisions as he struggled through his final stages of cancer, she found out rather quickly that she had the wrong conception of both family and autonomy. The autonomy practiced in the Eritrean culture of the young man was markedly different than she had thought. It was through his telling and her listening about the fabric of this man's "family" that Marianne learned a new way of conceiving of "family." Not only was autonomy extended beyond himself as a patient, but the notion of family was dramatically different. One of the important decision makers in his case was a stranger to the patient. The patient and his genetic family wanted Marianne to grant equal weight and credibility to this stranger as a member of his family, making decisions on behalf of the patient.

The focus on narrative highlights the character of the participants in the story. The actors in the story portray characters of a certain sort. Almost any story has good guys and bad guys; persons with virtue and persons with vice. And so we turn to what is called "virtue" or "character-based" approaches to religion and ethics.

Virtue ethics

The way of virtue is usually intimately connected to religion and spirituality, though it is true that one need not be either to be virtuous. Religion and spiritual practices shape human character traits more effectively throughout history than most other human institutions. One of the ways the virtues accomplish this is through the practice of upholding an exemplar to mimic and model. Traditions within every one of the world's religions routinely appeal to moral and religious exemplars. Indeed, it would be virtually impossible to imagine Christianity without Jesus, Islam without Muhammad, or Buddhism without Siddhartha. Those of us charged with imbuing the religious values and convictions of a faith tradition use reinforcing techniques to encourage our children to behave as our religious heroes have in the past. And again, this sort of reinforcement method is not limited to religion. You may recall the old Nike brand shoe commercials that said, simply, "I want to be like Mike" (Sommers and Sommers 2004: 209–276).

This character-based approach has bearing on both sides of any clinical religious scenario. The patient and the patient's family and friends do well when they practice the virtues of courage, insight, openness, and vulnerability. Similarly, there are key virtues that caregivers practice so as to provide the best possible healthcare to patients and their families. According to physician-philosopher Edmond Pellegrino, fortitude, compassion, integrity, practical reason, and self-effacement, among others, are essential to remain true to the history of both healthcare and religion (Pellegrino and Thomasma 1993). To single out one virtue prevalent in religious communities that is essential to caregiving in our view, we will highlight self-effacement or altruism below.

Virtues are not easily developed or perfected. Some believe that our personal character traits are primarily genetic rather than something that one can learn, practice, or perfect. Character traits like open-mindedness or stubbornness seem to be things we come by naturally, whereas virtues like compassion and courage are qualities we may learn and practice over time (Borba 2002). Indeed, at the outset of learning a virtue like courage, we may have to fake it (Herdt 2008: 23–32). In a stressful situation, we may be scared to death, but externally no observer would be able to discern that about us. Internal motivation and disposition are essential to the authentic exercise of the virtues. An external observer cannot tell when they see me engage in an apparently compassionate act whether or not I am actually compassionate. A duty-based perspective on the life of faith stresses that one engages in an act that God or the gods have demanded. When I compassionately help an old person across the street, you may see me as a virtuous person, but I may simply be doing my duty according to my interpretation of what God requires. This is not the way of virtue. The way of virtue calls for personal authenticity and consistent, practiced intention to care for others out of the compassion in your heart and soul. Habituating such character is the way of virtue, and religion is part and parcel of any such habituation.

There are many influences of personal development for those seeking religious and character growth in the way of virtue. Yes, one's genetics makes a difference. So also, the family, friends, and communities within which one is raised make an immense difference. Healthcare itself has a certain cluster of virtues that are emphasized and practiced throughout the education and professional development of caregivers at every level of patient care. One of the most important virtues in the history of healthcare professionalism is called altruism. Altruism is the prioritizing of the needs of the other (in this case, the patient) over one's own needs. In this relational orientation, matters of consequence, duty, and even virtue become lost in the intensity and importance of the caring. In the past 50 years or so, this attention to relationships has come to be known as "care ethics."

Care ethics

The care ethic demands that the primary concern of religion and the moral life is the relationship among all involved parties. If, for instance, I am pondering whether or not to lie to someone who asks me how I like their new tie, a care ethic founded upon the relationship I have with this person would prioritize the depth and details of that relationship over any sense of duty or concern for consequences. To use a more difficult example, if I held deep moral convictions that abortion should never be allowed and my closest friend asked me to accompany her to an abortion clinic for emotional care and support, a care orientation to religion and spirituality may compel me to go with her.

But what is it about the relationships with others that provides such a strong orientation to clinical interactions with patients? Traditionally, relational or caring aspects of patient interactions are associated with nursing. Nurses are the warm, fuzzy, caring ones while medical doctors and surgeons are the technicians who do the hard analysis and decision making. Curing aspects of patient interactions are traditionally associated with physicians (Jecker 2004: 371). With the present-day ascendance of a more relational approach to medical care, this traditional dynamic is breaking down and should continue to do so.

One central teaching of the care ethic is to realize and act upon the fact of human interdependence as opposed to human independence and individualism. As Nel Noddings puts it in the introduction to the second edition of her seminal work, "Virtually all care theorists make the relational more fundamental than the individual" (Noddings 2013). All individual actions have immense ripple effects in the lives of others in relationship to the person. Recognizing and accounting for this interdependence is essential. The force of personal autonomy is somewhat blunted by this emphasis if autonomy is taken to be atomistic and individualized. And the extent and influence of one's personal moral actions are highlighted in this approach. Again, the point here is not to completely discount other elements important to religion and the moral life, but to prioritize relationships with others. To additionally highlight the narrative approach to religion, a care approach wants to account for the influence of the story of one's life and relationships.

A narrative approach is an important element of a robust concern for others in a relationship-based religious life. If the stories that you and your family have always told about abortion, for instance, are condemnatory then the request from your friend to accompany her will make for a particularly difficult decision. On the other hand, if those stories have always sought to extend understanding and grace, then you will be more positively disposed toward attending to your friend.

Further, when someone is hospitalized, those of us who care for patients realize our care is extended to that patient's family precisely because of the relationships within that family. Those relationships may be functional or dysfunctional, pleasant or unpleasant, but we intuitively recognize this important approach to the manner with which we reach out to the family.

Let this focus on the interdependence of our moral lives launch us into our final concern, namely, how we manage our religion in relation to the religions of those we care for in clinical healthcare. Historically, religion and politics are topics that we all agree not to fight about. In healthcare, particularly in pluralist America, we enter a world where our interactions with others of different faiths challenge us daily. What do we make of this challenge? What are the key areas of religious instruction on ethics and morality that enable us to honor and respect all persons we care for?

Religion and spirituality

It has become increasingly common in contemporary Western culture to distinguish between religion and spirituality. Religion is typically associated with the belief systems and practices of established faith traditions. Spirituality, in contrast, is typically associated with the personal search for meaning of individuals. Of course, one's personal spirituality may be linked to a religious tradition. But in many of today's cultures, the linkage between individual spiritual journeys and organized religious traditions has been diminished. For our purposes in this chapter, we note this distinction, but we have chosen to include both religion and spirituality in our discussion of spiritually nurturing and respectful patient care.

Perceptive healthcare professionals often notice their patients' faith or spirituality can be among their most important resources for coping with serious illness or injury. Failure to take these resources into account represents less than optimal care for many patients. On the other hand, spiritual care of patients who may come from many different faith traditions, as well as those who would benefit from spiritual attention but have no identifiable religious commitments, requires following some carefully chosen norms. Here, we discuss five such guides for compassionate care (Winslow and Wehtje-Winslow 2007: 63–66):

1   Understand the patient's religious needs and resources.
2   Follow the expressed wishes of the patient, to the extent this is feasible.
3   Do not prescribe or pressure patients to adopt new practices or convictions.
4   Do not proscribe the patient's religious practices or resources.
5   Understand your own religious convictions, practices, and resources.

Understand the patient's religious needs and resources

Most of us live in highly pluralistic cultures when it comes to religion and spirituality. This means that no single faith tradition or religious vision will have dominance. Given this reality, it is important to permit patients to self-identify whatever they wish to have known about their spiritual needs and resources. Non-intrusive conversations that welcome such exploration are best facilitated in a context that carefully avoids stereotyping based on a patient's apparent ethnicity or perceived cultural heritage. People differ. And even within a named faith tradition, there may be a wide range of personal beliefs and practices. All of the major religions have numerous, distinctive iterations of their faith. We suggest finding thoughtful ways to welcome patients' expression of their own spiritual journey and its significance at this point in their lives. We offer the following script as one example of a way to open such a conversation: "Faith is often important to people when they need healthcare. Is there anything you want us to know about your faith or spiritual practices that might be helpful in your care?"

The hope is to open a pathway of discovery with the patient. No particular script will be suitable for all occasions, all patients, or all caregivers. A better method is for the caregiver to develop an approach with which he or she feels confident. The goal of such conversations is to help the patient identify her or his own spiritual resources and then permit the patient to express to caregivers how these resources may be helpful in planning for the best possible care. The purpose of these conversations should not be an attempt to bring about a patient's conversion to a new religious tradition.

Follow the expressed wishes of the patient, to the extent this is feasible

As noted earlier, it is often difficult to find the best balance among the principles of respecting the patient's autonomy, providing significant health benefits, and avoiding harm to the patient. Traditionally, the practice of medicine has been shaped by the expectation of paternalism, or the belief that the important decisions about the patient's care should be made unilaterally by the healthcare professionals, especially the physician in charge. After all, it is the physician who is expected to have the greatest knowledge of the science and art of medical care. So whose judgment should govern when caregivers perceive that the patient's beliefs, decisions, and practices may be harmful to his or her health? This question may be peculiarly perplexing when the patient, influenced by strongly held religious beliefs, makes decisions that seem inimical to the usual goals of healthcare. Those goals were usually informed by clinical considerations that had little, if anything, to do with the patient's religious convictions. Learning to navigate the caregiving territory that includes clinical goals of the healthcare team, the personal spiritual goals of the patient, and the established norms of society requires artfulness, creativity, and balance. In finding the balance, it is the settled ethical conviction of our society that we begin with the competent patient's expressed wishes.

The priority our culture gives to patient autonomy is tempered, however, by the professional responsibilities of healthcare providers to offer only those reasonable treatment alternatives for which there is adequate evidence. Healthcare professions are never required to offer or to provide treatment alternatives that, in their professional judgment, are unwarranted in light of scientific evidence. It is imperative for caregivers to maintain personal integrity within the boundaries of their professional knowledge and ethical commitments. If the values of caregivers and care recipients clash, honest attempts to preserve the personal integrity of all those involved can help to reduce moral distress. Such distress may arise from a dissonance of values in a variety of healthcare settings. Specifically, religious convictions sometimes do generate conflicts associated with relatively high levels of distress. Occasionally, such distress may be ameliorated by the caregiver's reassignment to care for other patients with whom there is no dissonance. Healthcare organizations have a wide range of policies that govern the degree to which conscientious objection is allowed as an acceptable option for caregivers. Such policies, in our experience, are rarely invoked. But, when needed, they can provide a useful means to manage distress and conflict.

Within this context of the balance of caring for one's self and for one's patients, a word about altruism is in order. Altruism is the purposeful placement of the needs of another person over one's own needs. Altruistic acts tend to flow from the actor's sense of compassion in relationship to the needs of others. Every major religion described in this book espouses the virtue of altruism. Today's healthcare would benefit from careful reflection on the importance of altruism. This is especially true in a culture that tends to emphasize self-gratifying actions, and less often highlights the essential role of altruism. One implication, in our view, is the altruistic willingness to find creative ways to accommodate the religious needs and respect the religious resources of patients and their families, even when this creates some discomfort for caregivers. A further implication is that caring for inpatients should never include prescribing that they adopt new religious practices or convictions.

Do not prescribe or pressure patients to adopt new practices or convictions

Caregivers interact with patients in a wide variety of settings, some of which may be conducive to conversations about religion, faith, spirituality, and personal practices. As a general rule, however, restraint should be exercised when it comes to introducing new religious ideas. This is all the more true as the critical nature of the patient's illness becomes more acute – despite oft-repeated stories of deathbed religious conversions. Even though some religious caregivers may be passionate about witnessing for their faith and desirous of helping patients share in that faith, such passion needs to be modulated by the realization that ours is a religiously pluralistic culture, and healthcare is not the proper setting for seeking religious converts.

Of course, it can happen that a patient will request information and insight from a religiously devout caregiver. Even so, an abundance of caution is in order. Patients are often extremely vulnerable when they are in critical need of care. And the caregiving context usually includes family members and friends of the patient. So conversations about faith are often not limited to the individual patient. Whole person care requires paying attention to the patient's social and familial realities. The insights of narrative ethics and care ethics, as mentioned earlier in this chapter, can be enlightening in this regard. They may make caregivers more aware of the stories within which the patients live their lives, including the final chapters of those lives. And they may enliven healthcare professionals' willingness to honor and respect the personal relationships that affect patients' lives.

Do not proscribe the patient's religious practices or resources

This is the complementary norm to that of forswearing the prescription of new religious practices and beliefs. Today's healthcare, governed as it is by many state and federal requirements, is highly controlled and monitored. Many healthcare facilities must forbid certain practices related to religion as it may be practiced in patients' homes or faith communities. For instance, the burning of candles is prohibited for safety reasons. Many hospitals have a "no fragrance" policy that forbids caregivers and families from engaging in the use of any essential oils or incense, thus ruling out some religious rituals as they are customarily practiced. This point came to the fore in a recent case in which one of the authors (Carr) was involved. A Hmong family's shaman came to the hospital to help care for a child. Though open to allowing for such involvement, the hospital had to forbid any ritual that entailed burning or smoke.

Additionally, though not necessarily related to religious practice, something as simple as bringing flowers to patients may be forbidden. Herbal products that some may use in the belief that they enhance health will normally have to be scrutinized by the hospital's pharmacists. Such natural remedies will likely need to be brought to the pharmacy in original packaging for inspection and approval before being allowed into use by the patient. Drug interactions with natural remedies are a relatively new and critical matter requiring caution as Western medicine and non-Western medicine come into the pluralistic mix of modern healthcare in America.

Understand your own religious convictions, practices, and resources

The human character trait of self-reflection is present in each of us at varying levels. Any person who can meaningfully say the words, "I said to myself," must understand that the "I" who is the agent can subject the "Me" to examination. Some of us practice this virtue more easily than others. The role of self-reflection is essential in clinical healthcare professionals to a high degree. All professionals may benefit from enhanced self-reflection. But what is nice for all professions can be a critical necessity for those professionals who care for patients in hospitals if the goal is genuine, whole-person care.

In common parlance, knowing one's self is essential to being open to knowing the Other. By knowing one's self we mean to emphasize the fact that exploration and expansion of our knowledge of the world's religions necessarily expands our sense of self. We cannot fully understand what others believe within a vacuum. When we learn what others believe we necessarily compare and contrast what we ourselves believe. This comparison and contrasting process can take a number of default perspectives. For instance, a person might say to her or himself, "nothing I might learn about another religion will ever affect the things I currently believe." Alternatively, a person might be so open to the beliefs of another such that nothing of one's present beliefs will remain intact – everything might be changed by exposure and subsequent adoption of the beliefs of the other. Historically, a well-established function in religious studies was that of apologetics and polemics. An apologist for a particular religious tradition takes every opportunity to defend the rightness of his or her faith while often attempting to demonstrate its superiority over the faith of others. Through polemical arguments, the religious beliefs and practices of other traditions are thus rejected and characterized as false and perhaps even demonic.

In our view, healthcare professionals may positively benefit from deep and abiding religious and spiritual convictions and practices, but they must refrain from engaging in apologetics or polemics in the clinical care of patients. Respectful relationships with patients and with caregiving colleagues require that such contentious approaches to religion or spirituality be set aside. Honesty about one's own convictions and a willingness to exercise humility in sharing them are essential to the ethical, compassionate practice of healthcare professionals.

Bibliography

Beauchamp, T. and Childress, J. (2013) *Principles of Biomedical Ethics*, 7th edn, New York: Oxford University Press.

Borba, M. (2002) *Building Moral Intelligence: The Seven Essential Virtues That Teach Kids to Do the Right Thing*, San Francisco: Jossey-Bass, A Wiley Imprint.

"Final Report to the European Commission on the Project, Basic Ethical Principles in Bioethics and Biolaw, 1995–1998." Available online at: https://ec.europa.eu/research/biosociety/pdf/final_rep_95_0207.pdf.

Hauerwas, S. and Jones, L. G., eds (1989) *Why Narrative: Readings in Narrative Theology*, Grand Rapids: Eerdmans.

Herdt, J. A. (2008) *Putting on Virtue: The Legacy of the Splendid Vices*, Chicago: University of Chicago Press.

Hunter, K. M. (2004) "Narrative," *Encyclopedia of Bioethics*, San Francisco: Macmillan Reference USA, Thompson Gale.

Jecker, N. (2004) "Care: Contemporary ethics of care," *Encyclopedia of Bioethics*, San Francisco: Macmillan Reference USA, Thompson Gale.

Jonsen, A. R. (1991) "Of balloons and bicycles – or – the relationship between ethical theory and practical judgment," *Hastings Center Report*, vol. 21, no. 5: 14–16.

Jonsen, A. R., Siegler, M., and Winslade, W. (2015) *Clinical Ethics: A Practical Approach to Ethical Decision Making in Clinical Medicine*, 8th edn, New York: McGraw-Hill Education/Medical.

Nelson, H. L. (1997) *Stories and Their Limits: Narrative Approaches to Bioethics*, New York: Routledge.

Noddings, N. (2013) *Caring: A Relational Approach to Ethics and Moral Education*, Los Angeles: University of California Press.

Pellegrino, E. and Thomasma, D. (1993) *The Virtues in Medical Practice*, New York: Oxford University Press.

Rawls, J. (1971) *A Theory of Justice*, Cambridge: Belknap of Harvard University Press.

Sommers, C. and Sommers, F. (2004) *Vice & Virtue in Everyday Life: Introductory Readings in Ethics*, 6th edn, Belmont, CA: Wadsworth/Thompson Learning.

UNESCO, "Universal Declaration of Bioethics and Human Rights." Available online at: http://unesdoc.unesco.org/images/0014/001461/146180E.pdf.

Winslow, G. and Wehtje-Winslow, B. (2007) "Ethical boundaries of spiritual care," *Medical Journal of Australia*, vol. 186, no. 10: S63–S66.

Suggested texts

Brody, H. (2002) *Stories of Sickness*, New York: Oxford University Press.

Gilligan, C. (1993) *In a Different Voice: Psychological Theory and Women's Development*, Cambridge, MA: Harvard University Press.

Hauerwas, S. (1981) *A Community of Character: Toward a Constructive Christian Social Ethic*, Notre Dame: University of Notre Dame Press.

Realin, A. gen. ed. (2012) *A Desk Reference to Personalizing Patient Care*, 3rd edn, Maitland, FL: Florida Health Publishing.

3 American Indian religions

Carla Gober and Roy Kim

Oh, Great Spirit, Whose voice I hear in the winds,
And whose breath gives life to all the world,
Hear me, I am small and weak, I need your strength and wisdom.
Let me walk in beauty and make my eyes ever behold the red and
    purple sunset.
Make my hands respect the things you have made and my ears sharp to
    hear your voice.
Make me wise so that I may understand the things you have taught
    my people.
Let me learn the lessons you have hidden in every leaf and rock.
I seek strength, not to be greater than my brother, but to fight my greatest
    enemy – myself.
Make me always ready to come to you with clean hands and straight eyes.
So when life fades, as the fading sunset, my Spirit may come to you
    without shame.
Native American Prayer, translated by Lakota Sioux Chief Yellow Lark
in 1887

Introduction

"You can come in now." The nurse encourages me into the room where my father is having basal cell skin cancer removed from his face. I am unprepared for the sight. There is a hole the size of a quarter in my father's nose where the physician has removed tissue. My father talks and jokes with me, seemingly unaware of the gaping hole. I feel queasy and excuse myself.

My mother joins me in the hall and states the facts simply. "The doctor is examining the tissue to see if he needs to remove more."

More? My mind races back and forth over the events that have brought us here. My father identifies himself as American Indian, of the Cherokee tribe. American Indian artwork lines the walls of one room in his home and he operates in the world with a spirituality and connectedness to all things, including animals and nature. He believes in "natural remedies." Up until the surgery, he wanted to treat the growing mysterious skin changes on his nose with herbs boiled into a thick paste. He applied the herb poultices to his face and later recounted stories of how the poultices "pulled out" the cancer. In one case, he froze the tissue that had been pulled out and used the frozen sample to illustrate his stories. He believed that his "cancer cream" only affected cancer cells, leaving normal skin unaffected. Over time the rest of us watched as the mysterious redness grew larger. Several times we pleaded with him to see a physician. Reluctantly, he consented.

My mother interrupts my thoughts. "The physician says that if we had waited much longer, it might have gone into his brain." As I walk back into the room, her comment helps me deal with my guilt that I am somehow responsible for his current disfigurement. For the next two months, my dad looks as if he has had a stroke. His mouth is asymmetrical due to nerve disruption. At one point, my father states that if he had to do it over, he would not go to the physician. He believes that God provided natural remedies for every kind of illness and that the herb poultices would have worked if just given time.

Eventually, the wound heals, the nerve returns to normal function and my father's skin looks perfect again, without asymmetry. But his mind is not changed. If the skin cancer returns, he will use the herb remedies. Soon after hearing of his decision, I happen upon an advertisement for a new basal cell skin cancer cream, derived of herbs. It affects only cancer cells, leaving normal skin unaffected.

I am stunned. Was my father correct? Was his concoction similar to the new medical cream in the advertisement? Was I wrong to insist that he get help from a physician? Does the positive outcome justify my insistence? My father did not see Western medicine as "the remedy." For him it was only one of several paths to healing, and not the most important one. Unlike my father, I saw Western medicine as the most important path to healing. We were each caught between two worlds.

My father does not represent every American Indian. He represents the complexities of those who identify as American Indian and of the deep connections between spirituality, nature, and healing. He also represents those whose worlds are not understood. When two different groups appreciate multiplicity and value knowledge that is outside their own sphere, rather than being *caught* between two worlds as my father and I were, they are "dancing between two worlds" (Gustafson 1997). The dance moves them both beyond perceptions of diametric opposition to a potentially creative space that enlarges the view of the world for both involved.

In healthcare clinics across North America, American Indians who enter the clinical world of "Western" medicine enter into this dance. As healthcare providers your ability to both understand and enter into this "dance" will enhance the healing enterprise in your clinic.

Demographics

The United States Census Bureau estimates that as of 2010 there are approximately 5.2 million people in the United States who identify themselves as

American Indian or Alaska Native (alone or in combination with other races), amounting to 1.7 percent of the total population (Norris et al. 2012). This estimate is projected to go up to 8.6 million within the next forty years and partially reflects the increasing numbers of people who identify themselves as American Indian (Passell 1996: 79–102).

The definition of "Indian" is complex. Many people, including the American Indians themselves, use the terms *American Indian* and *Native American* interchangeably, thus the terms are used interchangeably in this chapter. However, the preferred term seems to be *American Indian*, with some desiring to be referred to according to the tribal group in which they belong (Bureau of Labor Statistics 1995). There are 562 federally recognized tribes and nations in the United States, with ten main American Indian tribal groups and four main Alaska Native groups (Indian Affairs n.d.). The main American Indian tribal groups are: Apache, Cherokee, Chippewa, Choctaw, Creek, Iroquois, Lumbee, Navaho, Pueblo, and Sioux. The main Alaska Native tribal groups are: Alaska Athabascan, Aleut, Eskimo, and Tlingit-Haida (US Census Bureau 2000). These tribes speak over 200 indigenous languages. This only begins to illustrate the diversity within the American Indian and Alaska Native groups. Thus, it is impossible to avoid generalizations that gloss over tribal differences. However, in general, a broader overview is important for basic knowledge.

Further complicating this is that not everyone who identifies as American Indian is actually counted as Indian. General guidelines have been developed to determine eligibility for health services. By some guidelines, an Indian is a person who has two qualifications: (1) ancestors living in America before its discovery, and (2) being recognized as Indian by his or her tribe or community (Cohen 1982). Using this protocol, my father would not be considered Indian, even though both parents are from Indian descent. He is not currently recognized as Indian by his tribe, simply because he has not initiated that recognition; however, *he identifies himself* as American Indian.

Two surveys shed light on Native American Religion. One is the National Survey of Religious Identification conducted in 1990 and the American Religious Identity Survey conducted in 2001. Both suggest that Native American Religion is among the top twenty (twelfth out of twenty) religions in the United States, with a 119 percent increase between 1990 and 2000, and representing 0.05 percent of the United States population in 2000. Demographics within Native American Religion are more complex. First, many Native Americans do not regard their spiritual beliefs as religion. There is no word for *religion* in the Native languages. Their religion is a way of life that integrates all aspects of life into a whole, and it is understood entirely within the context of the spiritual and the sacred. Thus, Native American religion and spirituality is entirely cultural. One does not "convert" to this religion any more than one "converts" to being Native American. Second, due to a history of long-term contact with missions and Christian influences, many Native Americans are Christian while also holding onto traditional tribal beliefs.

History

One of the first treaties between the United States and Indians was made in 1778 between the United States on one side and Captain White Eyes, Captain John Kill Buck, and Captain Pipe on the other. It was a treaty established for the purposes of peaceful passage through Indian Territory and to assure the Indians that there was no intent to "take possession of their country." Article I states that "All offences or acts of hostilities by one, or either of the contracting parties against the other, be mutually forgiven, and buried in the depth of oblivion, never more to be had in remembrance" (*Treaty with the Delawares: 1778*, Yale Law School n.d.). It was about respect and possession. What was not understood at the time by those marking "x" as their signatures, or by those who could write, was that this Article about respect and possession was only the beginning of devastation for the American Indian. Treaty-making ended by 1871, and from 1887 to 1934 the United States government promoted assimilation by prohibiting American Indian ceremonies and promoting English boarding school education.

In 1822, Jedediah Morse published a report for the purposes of "awakening the attention ... to the state of this neglected and oppressed people" by counting Indians and identifying where they lived (Morse 1822: 9). The real awakening should have come with the disease and death taking place by the mid-1800s. Smallpox killed thousands of Indians, in some cases wiping out entire groups. According to Henry Rowe Schoolcraft, "Language, however forcible, fails to give an idea of the reality" (Schoolcraft 1857). By the end of the nineteenth century, there were approximately 250,000 American Indians (estimates of the population at the time of European encroachment range between 1.2 and 12 million).

In 1921, through the Bureau of Indian Affairs, the federal government encouraged the use of force to halt religious practices that would hinder assimilation, but by 1928, the assimilation project was declared a failure and religious and cultural practices were soon considered legal. In the 1970s, the US government returned some sacred lands to the American Indians (a sacred lake to the Taos Pueblo Indians and a portion of Mount Adams to the Yakama Indians), but struggles for religious freedoms continued through the 1980s and 1990s over issues such as control of sacred lands, exercise of religious and cultural practices prohibited by other laws (substances used in ceremonies etc.), the protection of knowledge (sacred and general) from exploitation, and the control of human remains and sacred objects held in museums.

When the Indians were relegated to vast tracts of land, the wound was not just to the American Indians themselves. In their minds, the earth was wounded, which meant that they as caretakers of the earth were also wounded at a very deep soul level. In relegating the American Indians to reservations, the US government assumed certain responsibilities, one of which was the provision of health services, but there was little understanding of the depth and spiritual nature of the wound (Rhoades 2000). By 1849, the Office of Indian Affairs dealt mostly with health on the reservations and provided minimal health services. By the beginning of the twentieth century, it seemed that the Indian population would continue to dwindle; however, within the second half of the twentieth century there was a fivefold increase in the population due to rising birth rates, declining mortality, increasing numbers of people identifying as American Indian and Alaska Native (who also identify themselves in other groups), and other factors (Rhoades 2000).

In 1955, the Indian Health Service (IHS) was established and now serves members of Indian tribes throughout the country. It also funds contracts, such as one in Southern California called the Riverside-San Bernardino County Indian Health, Inc. (RSBCIHI), which is a tribally managed healthcare organization comprised of a consortium of ten tribes. Among the goals of RSBCIHI are to provide culturally appropriate healthcare services by respecting and abiding by customs and traditions and to promote wellness by striving to provide state-of-the-art healthcare. Through this complex organization of community-oriented primary care, American Indians receive basic healthcare. One of the challenges is that, while Indians are eligible for this care, many move away from the reservations into metropolitan areas and reside outside the scope of IHS and tribal care systems (Snipp 2000: 56). Currently, the comprehensive health service delivery system of the IHS agency serves 2.2 million patients constituting approximately 70 percent of the American Indians and Alaska Natives. This number represents those who reside in or near reservations where IHS services are available (US Department of Health and Human Services 2015).

Another factor complicates healthcare delivery. The Indian elder is a position of leadership based on wisdom, community service, and experience, rather than chronological age. The community group may refer to someone as young as forty or in their early fifties as an "elder." They are the ones most closely connected to a painful historical past on one hand, and the heroic oral histories on the other. They are the keepers of the sacred songs that often are not allowed to be taped and studied by outsiders. The younger generations sometimes go to them for health remedies, either before seeking medical care or after Western modern medicine has failed. In contrast, from the perspective of the Indian Health Service, an Indian elder is someone fifty-five years of age or older. For healthcare givers within the IHS, Indian elders are simply the aging group within the American Indian population – older versions of the young, rather than keepers of a rich tradition (Deloria 1997).

The term "tribal sovereignty" suggests that Indian tribes/nations have the authority to govern themselves, which means that, in general, the states have no legal jurisdiction in Indian country, or reservation territory. Indian tribes can make laws affecting conduct, enforce laws through tribal police, exclude non-members from the reservation, and regulate environmental protection. This idea of sovereignty creates complexities in the way Indians relate to the federal government on issues connected to healthcare (Kim 2008).

Beliefs and practices

General

Indians have a different way of thinking when they are within traditional cultural contexts and natural environments, notes Donald Fixico, a leading American Indian historian. He argues that Indian thinking is "visual and circular in philosophy," suggesting that it is a combination of two realities – the physical and the metaphysical (Fixico 2003: xii). Decision making is a response to listening and observing the natural environment and then balancing all factors in the process of coming to a consensus. "The right decision is the best decision for all concerned" (Fixico 2003: xii). Of particular interest is the concept of "listening" and "seeing." "Listening" has less to do with sounds than with gaining information for understanding the connections and their meanings. "Seeing" is visualizing all the possible connections and their relationships with each other. It is viewing from a holistic perspective. For example, with my father's skin cancer, my primary concern was his nose, and whether or not the skin changes were actually cancer. For my father, it had more to do with his life, his desire to know the actual medical diagnosis (or not to know it), his relation to nature and natural healing, how the current moment might play out in the future, and the process of making a decision. For him it was about the whole, and all the connections that go with that. Thus, "seeing" and "listening" make up Indian thinking.

With the circular way of thinking found in the Indian mind, there are not two focal points; there is only one, and all illustrations reflect on that one point with the purpose of increasing understanding and the possibility for harmony. The non-Indian mind is more linear, proceeding from point A to point B and valuing empirical evidence more highly than the story. In linear thinking, the purpose is to pursue goals, work hard, look to the future, and not be distracted by those around you.

Circular thinking is all about the capacity to look in all directions and appreciate everything that one sees. At the center of this circle is peace – a sacred space of rest, balance, and wholeness that defies the chaos going on around it. Sickness is being out of balance, of failing to see the connections, of having no peace at the center. In this way, religion and medicine connect. Both address issues of balance, harmony, and wholeness. While most American Indians have been educated in mainstream schools, many still "see" from this indigenous non-linear perspective and this has implications for healthcare (Fixico 2003: xii).

While this form of thinking does characterize the Indian "mindset" in general, each tribe is different, each is unique. In comparison to the typical North American mindset, however, Indians can be said to consider life to be sacred. Some feel themselves to be "holy people" and to be "called to live a holy life." Rituals and ceremonies are essential, as are those who conduct them. These shaman or "medicine men (or women)" also help the community to maintain traditional healing practices. Oral traditions remain strong, thus there is no written scripture in their religions. Relationship with the land is very important to most American Indians, which is deeply related to the experience of religion. In the end, at death, Indians often believe they "go to God."

Some Native American beliefs are more universal, such as reverence and respect for life and the belief that all things are sacred – even rocks, plants, and dust. Another belief shared by most tribes is that death is a part of life and is not the result of an angry God (or other deity), but happens to all people once they have fulfilled the purpose for life. Another common belief is that to be healthy is to be in balance – mind, body, and spirit. Other beliefs are unique to the particular tribe of American Indians. Some tribes have restrictions on what they can look at. Some believe in ghosts, while others do not. Many tribes practice a similar ceremony, such as the sun dance, while practicing it differently.

What the tribes share is the belief in the sacredness of all things and people. While not all tribes describe themselves as a "holy people," they share the belief that their lives are infused with the spiritual – that life is about balance and the connection of all things. A common Lakota salutation and saying at the end of a prayer illustrates this respect and connectedness of all things – *Mitakuye Oyasin*, meaning "to all my relations," which includes family, extended family, and nature as well. People, mountains, and bodies of water are all sacred beings and make up the family, about which the American Indian cares deeply (Sutton and Nose 2005).

There are a variety of ceremonies and rituals. Some tribes allow children to be present during healing rituals (Lakota), believing that friends and family help restore the ill to balance, and some do not allow the presence of children (Apache). The purpose of the medicine men and women is to counteract the supernatural forces as much as possible. They refer to those who practice indigenous healing that focuses on physical healing, spiritual healing or both (Sutton and Nose 2005). These traditional healers understand the connections between nature and health and often use ceremonies to determine the cause and treatment of disease. These ceremonies can take up to several days (Spector 2000). Natural or traditional remedies include the use of herb medicines, special rituals, and sweat lodges (heated dome-shaped structures in which Indians have spiritual experiences). The use of traditional remedies illustrates the sense of connectedness with the natural world and the belief that one should live in harmony with it.

Some songs and prayers that accompany the ceremonies are secret, and those who know the songs must be present for the ceremonies to take place. This highlights the importance of the oral tradition of the Native American. The oral tradition begins with the telling of various creation stories, depending on the tribal tradition. Stories vary from an androgynous creator figure (for Zunis), to a stronger twin brother (many Native American cultures), or to a suffering hero figure (for Navajos). Among most tribes, however, there is the sense of a single creative force, which manifests itself in everything human and non-human. That creative force grants spirit-power to animals and other non-human entities. The stories also explore the notion of four directions, which must be in balance for health to be possible.

Native American myths contain all types of genres, including trickster myths such as Coyote and Iktome, who bring forth humans, while at the same time causing problems for them. This commitment to the oral tradition helped to preserve knowledge. It also preserved a flexibility that allowed the Native American to survive a variety of threats by integrating foreign aspects without losing itself.

American Indians are often passionate about protecting "Mother Earth" because she is "life itself." This religious or spiritual regard for the land typifies the way in which the American Indian connects with space rather than the more typical time-orientation of most Americans. It also suggests that while many Native Americans may be Christian, they often still connect to native spirituality. American Indians in general, regardless of the tribe or perspectives on Christianity, believe in the sacredness of the land – both general and particular. All land is sacred in that they are to live in harmony with it and not destroy it. In addition, particular lands are sacred in that American Indians have a particular commitment to take care of *that* land – to fish and hunt with ethical commitments to the moral standing of all that lives within it. Traditionally, the Native American communicated with the Creator through interacting with the natural elements of animals, plants, and nature in general. Many were given symbolic animals (names, symbols) to reflect their own human characteristics, or with the hopes that these animal spirits would infuse their animal characteristics into the Indian. In this way, fishing, hunting, religion, and the land are all interconnected in ways that are inseparable.

In conclusion, to understand Native American beliefs and practices, we must "listen" and "see" through non-linear thinking rather than linear, empirical thinking. To accomplish this, narrative and storytelling are the preferred methods for the discussion, as well as exploring a variety of metaphors. In the introduction to his book, *Healing the Soul Wound*, Eduardo Duran, himself an American Indian and a psychologist working in Indian territory, explains that he faced the decision of whether to "embroider the fabric of the clinical work with academic language and theoretical constructs or simply say what needs to be said" (Duran 2006: 1). In the end, he decided simply to present the story. If we listen well, it may be necessary to modify or change some Western practices in order to better serve the American Indian population (Duran 2006).

Health and disease

Keith is a thirty-two-year-old American Indian man who lives in an urban area and works as a salesman in a small hobby shop during the day and as a cabinetmaker in the evening. He has little contact with his Indian culture, occasionally participating in cultural events on a reservation located an hour's drive from where he lives. During a visit to his local physician for a diabetes check-up, he confesses that he is struggling with alcohol and wonders if he is depressed. He tells the story of picking up his gun and holding it to his chest, imagining that all the pain in his life is over. Laughingly he states, "Maybe I should get some bee stingers from the Elder. Maybe that would help."

In order to understand and address Keith's situation, some background will help. American Indians and Alaska Natives living in the United States have a lower health status than the average American. They have lower life expectancy by 4.4 years (73.7 years compared to 78.1 for the average American) (Indian Health Service 2016) and higher infant mortality rates (7.61 out of 1,000 deaths compared to 7.0 out of 1,000 deaths) (Mathews et al. 2015). Table 3.1 shows the 1989–1991 and 2002–2004 mortality rates for specific disease processes as they compare with all races in the United States (Huff and Kline 1999: 281).

There are higher rates of some sexually transmitted diseases such as gonorrhea and syphilis (Centers for Disease Control and Prevention 2011). The leading cause of death in those aged 10–34 is unintentional injury, the second leading cause of death (ages 10–34) is suicide; the third is homicide. In those aged 45–85, the first and second leading causes of death are malignant neoplasms and heart disease, depending on the age (Centers for

Table 3.1 American Indian mortality rates for specific diseases compared with all races in the US

Disease	% greater 1989–1991	% greater 2002–2004
Tuberculosis	440	750
Alcoholism	430	550
Diabetes	154	190
Homicide	50	100
Suicide	43	70

Disease Control and Prevention 2013). In relation to mental health services, there is lack of funding and a high turnover of mental health professionals, and the mental health services are often not culturally appropriate. For these reasons, mental health services are often underutilized (Gone 2004: 10–18).

This background helps us understand Keith better. Given the tendency not to utilize mental health services, he confesses his psychological issues to his physician. Suicide is the second leading cause of death in his age category, with unintentional injury being the first, so his thoughts of suicide should not surprise us. He has little connection to his Indian culture, so in some ways he is disconnected from his past, and perhaps experiences disconnection in general, enhancing the feeling of depression.

Keith brings more than personal depression. He brings with him generations of stories related to suffering. The relation between historical events and current constructions of health/illness is both relevant and complex in the healing encounter. The concept of intergenerational trauma has been addressed widely in the literature. This concept suggests that the trauma that is not dealt with in a previous generation is passed down to the next generation to deal with, and may become more severe as it passes down (Nebelkopf and Phillips 2004). This trauma may be internalized and expressed as domestic and/or institutional violence. The American Indian considers historical trauma, or intergenerational trauma, as a wound to the soul or spirit, referred to by some as a "soul wound," giving it "spiritual dimensions" (Duran 2006). In this sense, Keith brings more than individual depression. He brings a historical context that is deeply connected to the soul or spirit, and this affects the clinical encounter.

Finally, while Keith has little connection to his Indian culture, it continues to inform him, and thus he explores the concept of traditional healing. Traditional healing practices often treat the person holistically, treating the physical body as well as the soul. His reference to a traditional healing practice suggests the ways in which Western and traditional healing practices may overlap. If Keith were to subscribe entirely to traditional practices, he might enter a formal ceremony for healing, with burning plants, throwing cornmeal, or using bee stingers to treat disease. What is less understood by the current physician is that while Keith questions the use of bee stingers as treatment, his deeper desire is that the current physician treats him from a holistic perspective – that his soul and his body are connected and unless his spirit is in harmony with the rest, little else matters.

Helping Keith manage his illness demands attention to many factors. The first is to the non-linear and narrative emphasis in the American Indian mindset. Emerging from his current sense of depression will require a new story. But before a new narrative can begin, the old one must be understood, and this involves understanding the "soul wound." In trying to understand the historical context, the practitioner can ask the following question: "Where did you learn how to do this?" This can be followed up with, "And where did *they* learn how to do this?"

The practitioner must also be aware of his or her own historical context and the complexities this might bring. In speaking of the American Indians, one female Caucasian physician stated, "Just by virtue of being Caucasian, I am sometimes initially viewed as the enemy." It is helpful when practitioners are in touch with and aware of their own woundedness. This also suggests that healing is not dependent on someone in a higher position or on the medical model itself, but that healing has something to do with understanding the dichotomy within one's self – a sort of harmonizing of opposites. Again, this idea undercuts the view that illness is simply a pathologized self and comes closer to a traditional Indian view that healing has to do with harmonizing various, even opposing, elements.

One's own historical context also affects transference which, in the world of the Indian, can be interpreted literally as energy transferring from one person to another – both negative and positive, depending on the practitioner's attitudes toward the Indian, and on whether one has worked out one's own personal history. If the practitioner is an American Indian, he or she must avoid the belief that by belonging to the same group, there is automatic understanding (Duran 2006).

Viewing the treatment of illness as a ceremony that has specific physical or metaphorical boundaries may also help move Keith toward a new, healthier story. For example, the office may be the "container" in which the healing ceremony takes place. Instead of smoke and cornmeal, there may be other objects with which an American Indian can identify – pictures, artwork, objects related to healing. Making a diagnosis is a part of this ceremony – the naming of illness. Identifying a diagnosis for the American Indian can be viewed as a type of naming ceremony, where spiritual identities accompany the name. For the American Indian, illness has its own consciousness and works out a purpose within the body to restore it to wholeness. It is not so much the goal to overcome illness as it is to have a relationship with it, to understand its purpose, and to harmonize with it. A diagnosis may not be perceived by the American Indian as something to "treat" or "conquer" as much as it is to be understood and harmonized. The root metaphor of illness for the Indian is closer to relationship than pathology (Duran 2006).

A useful model for such clinical interactions has been developed by Lakota tribal leader Gene Thin Elk. He has designed an indigenous, culturally specific model called *The Red Road to Recovery*, which has helped thousands of people toward the creation of a healthier personal story. This model works from a holistic perspective and incorporates many traditional practices that make healing relevant and sensitive to the needs of the American Indian population. This reconnecting of American Indians to their cultural background takes seriously an important and essential past. Rather than teaching the Indian how to be more Westernized, the model suggests that the healthcare practitioner must learn to speak Red (Nebelkopf and

Phillips 2004). Learning to speak Red might mean becoming familiar with local resources that are sensitive to the needs of the American Indian. It might also mean incorporating such resources into one's own practice.

It is important to note the degree to which American Indians identify with their traditional culture. Knowing whether they live on a reservation and the degree of belief in and contact with traditional practices is important. Keith is not unusual. Diabetes and depression are major health problems among American Indians. What surprises the physician is that when Keith attempts to describe the cause of his diabetes, in a quiet gentle voice he begins to reflect on the history of the American Indian, rather than on his personal history. According to him, his people have left the old ways of healing and adopted the foods of the White world and this is why he has diabetes. He explains his attempts to eat more traditional foods. What has previously appeared to the physician as non-compliance is actually a man trying to come to terms with his own history. He attempts to be connected to the past, and to restore it.

The American Indian's (re-)claiming of traditional foods and dietary taboos can take different forms, depending on the tribe and tradition. Traditionally, the issue has not been about what foods one is allowed to eat, but rather a focus on foods that create *wicozani* (Sioux word) or balance. Processed meats, sugared drinks, the lack of fresh produce, and easy access to drugs and alcohol have contributed to many and various health problems among American Indians, such as diabetes, obesity, and substance abuse. Following the medicine wheel, which has four sections representing the four natural elements, they seek balance among four food types – water, meat, gathered plants, and cultivated plants, which should be consumed in equal portions. When one returns to a more traditional way of eating in such a manner, balance and healing can occur.

The juxtaposition between the traditional and the modern can also be seen in the area of procreation and sexual morality. As with other attitudes, Native American attitudes about contraception have a history. Native American women have had hundreds of years of experience using natural, traditional contraceptive methods, such as not having sex during the most fertile times, using crushed roots of red cedar and juniper plants in teas, or making concoctions from other plants to prevent births, some of which are used in commercial products for oral contraceptives (Mexican wild yam). American Indians have also used plant substances to induce abortions and cause sterility. As for the use of commercial contraceptives, Native American women's attitudes vary. Many do not use them, influenced by their husbands, extended family, or historical concerns. In general, tribal traditions tend to work against the use of commercial contraceptives, although this is changing and is partially dependent on a woman's age and number of children.

On the issue of abortion, Native American traditional health practices include the use of plants (black cohosh, black snakeroot, and squaw root) to stimulate the uterus, cause menstruation, or induce abortion. Native American cultures also believe that family planning is a part of respecting Mother Earth, with many Native American women feeling that decisions for abortion lay within their sphere, instead of the sphere of men or governmental agencies or laws. At the same time, because of the sacred value that they place upon the life cycle that begins and continues through conception and pregnancy and the preference that they have for natural and traditional means, American Indians have generally been averse to the invasive abortion procedures carried out in Western clinical settings, leading some tribes to ban modern abortion procedures altogether from clinics on Indian reservations.

Not surprisingly, those in the modern Western world are not as familiar with the value of connections with the past. American Indian *connection* suffers from dislocation from native lands, weakened parental influence due to mission and boarding schools, and weakened cultural ties. The healthcare professional should explore ways to re-establish these protective factors. For example, Lakota children are *wakanheja* or sacred, and taking care of these children is a sacred responsibility for both parents and the community (Nebelkopf and Phillips 2004). The idea of family may not only refer to the nuclear family, but may often extend to clans and lineages, revealing systems of loyalties that are critical. In this way, the community joins together to take care of its own. Putting the American Indian back in contact with his or her own cultural values of connection are more important that trying to instill "modern" values.

Death and dying

According to one American Indian myth, death exists because Coyote prevented the chief medicine man from catching death (portrayed as a whirlwind) so death continues to roam the earth. While this would seem to make death fearful, few American Indians fear death because of their belief that all things are interdependent. American Indians view death as a journey that proceeds beyond death, with ancestral spirits returning to interact with the living. It is a natural part of life.

While most tribes believe in a spiritual journey to the afterlife, some have a fear of ghosts (Navajo and Apache), while others do not (Hopi). The Apache believe that the spirit hangs around after death and a person can get "ghost sickness" by touching a dead body. The Alaska Native has no conception of a supreme spirit, although ancestral spirits may come to the family. Others suggest that disease-causing agents can take the form of snakes or owls and enter our dreams, creating havoc or causing illness. Most tribes believe that illness might be incurred from handling a deceased body. Some remain present while a loved one is dying; others do not. Some tribes tie prayer feathers to the hair and each foot of the deceased to aid them in their journey to the afterlife.

While the suicide rates are high for American Indians, the traditional belief does not support it, suggesting that those who commit suicide wander aimlessly on the earth (Cox 2003). In one study of American Indians living on reservations, a strong protective factor against suicide was tribal spiritual orientation, or forms of spirituality derived from traditions that predate European contact (referred to as "cultural spirituality") (Garroutte et al. 2003: 1571–9). Traditional healing practices look at a person holistically, thus they address the soul as well as the physical body. When American Indians seek traditional health practices it may be this holistic perspective that they desire, and this perspective is often missing in Western medicine. Where the American Indian understands the connection between a troubled soul and a diseased body, Western medicine often denies, or at least fails to address, this connection.

Funeral concerns vary from tribe to tribe. Some tribes (Navajo) shun the body and effects of the deceased, believing that the ghost stays behind. They believe that the body should be buried quickly, while a wake may last for several days (called "sings"). Other tribes (Lakota) believe that the body can be held for a period of time before burial. Since families are matriarchal, generally it is the wife, mother, or grandmother of the deceased who makes the arrangements for burial. The family may want to transport the body to the home of the deceased and paint the face according to the tribe. Burial and cremation are both allowed, depending on the tribe. Sometimes family and friends help dig the grave, referred to as "The Dig."

At the funeral ceremony, often an elder presides and a funeral director is not involved at all. The ceremony may include drumming and singing, and a feast in honor of the deceased, and may continue through the night(s). Many Native Americans place personal items belonging to the deceased, such as clothes and blankets, in the grave. There is the belief that everything made has the spirit of the maker in it, thus they often cut or break the item to release that spirit. For this reason, often broken pottery surrounds the gravesite. Sometimes, even the end of the casket is left unsealed in order to allow the spirit to be released.

After the funeral is grief and, according to Native American culture, there are many lessons about grief, its duration, and what can grow out of grief. In the Shoshone legend of the Caterpillar People, a dying caterpillar man leaves behind a grieving caterpillar woman. She grieves for a year until Great Mystery tells her that it is time to stop, at which point she turns into a butterfly and brings the world beauty, grace, and color.

The most important thing is that those who help Native American families plan funerals need to respect Native traditions and work in cooperation with their spiritual leaders. Native Americans approach death with awe, reverence, and love for the departed, as well as a fear that knowledge about their beliefs may be used to their disadvantage, thus there may be some reticence on the subject. It would be helpful for the healthcare practitioner to understand this.

Conclusion

For the healthcare practitioner to treat patients such as Keith, there must be some understanding of his culture and religion, as well as his historical context. This takes time, which is why trust is not quickly or easily built. Keith's healthcare practitioner can treat him without fully understanding him, but the treatment will never approach what is necessary for Keith to find true healing. Keith's pain is larger than his current context. The naming of his "disease" will not be captured by the terms "diabetic" or "suicidal" or "depression." His disconnection will not be remedied by a prescription for medication. As is true in the case of my father, "next time" he may do something different. With Keith, there may not even be another "next time." To speak in the language of the American Indian is not just to make the notation of "American Indian" on the chart; it is to understand that the notation represents an entire history, a rich tradition, a deep connection with the land, a tradition of storytelling, and the infusion of sacredness in everything from children to the natural elements. To speak in the language of the American Indian is to realize the breadth and depth of

Table 3.2 Dos and don'ts

Dos	Don'ts
1 Recognize that illness and health are spiritually oriented and not just physiological pathology.	1 Do not treat the patient like a number; a creature present in your clinic that needs something you can give.
2 As the caregiver, try to allow yourself a deep and present emersion into your own sense of what it means to be a whole, unitive person who is ill. Be a "wounded healer."	2 Do not allow yourself to slide into a cold, detached technician.
3 Create and fully incorporate as many ways as possible of connecting with the patient. Include the use of the creative arts, metaphors, storytelling, dreams, and play.	3 Do not maintain those elements of your practice that put distance between you and your patient.
4 Effective connection must include understanding the story the patient has to tell. Stick with it, listen to it, and hear it.	4 Do not allow yourself to be distracted. When you are with your patient, be fully present.
5 In this connection, a kind of ceremonial connection, work with the patient to identify and name the illness.	5 Do not foist upon the patient a technical and complicated diagnosis. Find and identify the illness without collaboration with the patient.
6 Begin then to create a new story that incorporates as much as possible the traditional, cultural ways to return the patient to health.	6 Do not rush out of the appointment. Providing culturally sensitive care sometimes takes more time than you expect.
	7 Do not demand to practice modern Western medicine without being influenced or taught by traditional healing ways.
	8 Do not avoid being touched by the individual and the historical story.

woundedness as well as healing, the value of circular thinking, and the importance of an inner core of peace and harmony. It is to ask, "Can you tell me more about...," not just for the purposes of understanding, but for the purposes of being taught.

Case study

My pager went off and I jumped to attention. My OB patient had arrived at the hospital in active labor. I had followed her throughout her pregnancy and when I arrived at the hospital her room was stuffed full of family members. Her mother and aunt were at the head of the bed, helping her breathe through her contractions. At the foot of the bed stood a traditional midwife, also her caregiver. My patient was very traditional and I wanted to do all I could to support her, so I welcomed her family and midwife in this special event. It was important that she deliver her child naturally and according to her Native American beliefs. Throughout the night, she gradually progressed and the baby looked great on the monitors. By 3 am the nurse informed me that she was feeling like she needed to push, so I quickly entered the delivery room, excited to be a part of this special event. Indeed, I determined she was ready to start pushing. I watched the monitor, saw a contraction coming. My patient's face quickly changed, expressing her intense pain. It was time to try her first push. The mom and aunt each held a foot and pulled her legs back. The midwife coached her on breathing and began to press on her abdomen. My courageous young mother pushed with each contraction. Wave after wave of contractions, she pushed and pushed. After an hour passed, my concern became intense. The baby had made little progress. The traditional midwife tried different positions but the baby still was not moving down the birth canal. I stared at the baby's heart rate on the monitor and noticed that the pattern was beginning to change. The baby's heart was showing the strain of a very slow delivery. My patient and her family saw the concern on my face. I told her, "If the heart rate keeps dropping, we are going to need to take her to the operating room for a C-section." Moments later, I grabbed a consent form for her to sign, but she refused. Exhausted and frustrated, she began to cry. My heart ached for her as I paused to hold her hand. About that time, the midwife spoke, announcing that the baby will come, we just needed to give her more time. The midwife began to press down on my patient's abdomen and manipulate her body in ways I was not familiar with. Honestly, at this point I just was not sure what to do, but I knew the baby's distress was critical and I felt like I should do something.

Questions for reflection

1   Should I let her perform these maneuvers on my patient? Could this harm the baby?

2   Will the patient and family get upset if I stop her?

3   Do I really respect her traditional ways when this is what it comes to?

4   Ultimately, I am responsible for my patient and the baby. How do I intervene and take action without disrespecting her beliefs? Does this even matter in this situation?

Glossary

American Indian/Native American   The Indians themselves as well as those who study, research, and write on American Indians use the terms interchangeably.

Mitakuye Oyasin   A common Lakota salutation and saying at the end of a prayer illustrates the respect for and connectedness of all things. Means literally, "to all my relations."

Story/storytelling   In the mind of the American Indian, the purpose of the story is to define, create, and understand reality. The story, storytelling, and folklore are primary elements in maintaining tradition, preserving knowledge, and protecting the truth of the past for the American Indian.

Sweat lodge or "inipi"   Generally it takes place in a hut or mostly enclosed area and water is poured over hot rocks so that steam rises, creating a sauna-like effect. It often occurs before and after all other ceremonies, or is used as a stand-alone ceremony to cleanse or purify.

Traditional healing   Traditional healing includes the traditions around health and illness not based on Western science but on tribal beliefs about how to live. Each tribe has its own methods and materials put to use in these traditional healing techniques.

Bibliography

Bureau of Labor Statistics (1995) *US Census Bureau Survey.* Available online at: www.census.gov/prod/2/gen/96arc/ivatuck.pdf (accessed October 20, 2008).

Centers for Disease Control and Prevention (2011) *Indian Health Surveillance Report – Sexually Transmitted Diseases 2011*, Atlanta, GA: US Department of Health and Human Services.

Centers for Disease Control and Prevention (2013) *Leading Causes of Death by Age Group, American Indian or Alaska Native Males – United States, 2013*, Atlanta, GA: Centers for Disease Control and Prevention and Indian Health Service.

Cohen, F. (1982) *Handbook of Federal Indian Law*, Charlottesville, VA: Michie Co.

Cox, G. (2003) "The Native American way of death," in Bryant, C. (ed.) *Handbook of Death and Dying: Volume Two: The Response to Death*, Thousand Oaks, CA: Sage Publications.

Deloria Jr., V. (1997) *Red Earth, White Lies: Native Americans and the Myth of Scientific Fact*, Golden, CO: Fulcrum Publishing.

Duran, E. (2006) *Healing the Soul Wound: Counseling with American Indians and Other Native Peoples*, New York: Teachers College Press.

Fixico, D. (2003) *The American Indian Mind in a Linear World*, New York: Routledge.

Garroutte, E., Goldberg, J., Herrell, R., and Manson, S. (2003) "Spirituality and attempted suicide among American Indians," *Social Science & Medicine*, vol. 56, no. 7: 1571–9.

Gone, J. (2004) "Mental health services for Native Americans in the 21st century United States," *Professional Psychology: Research and Practice*, vol. 35: 10–18.

Gustafson, F. (1997) *Dancing Between Two Worlds: Jung and the Native American Soul*, New York: Paulist Press.

Huff, R. and Kline, M. (1999) *Promoting Health in Multicultural Populations: A Handbook for Practitioners*, Thousand Oaks, CA: Sage Publications.

Indian Affairs (n.d.) Available online at: www.doi.gov/bia/ (accessed November 22, 2008).

Indian Health Service (2016) *The Federal Health Program for American Indians and Alaska Natives*. Available online at: www.ihs.gov/newsroom/factsheets/disparities (accessed June 1, 2016).

Kim, R. (2008) Personal visit at the Morongo Indian Reservation, San Bernardino County, California, November 21, 2008.

Mathews, T. J., MacDorman, M. F., and Thoma, M. E. (2015) "Infant mortality statistics from 2013 period linked birth/infant death data set," *National Vital Statistics Reports*, vol. 64, no. 9, Hyattsville, MD: National Center for Health Statistics.

Morse, J. (1822) *A Report to the Secretary of War of the United States on Indian Affairs 1822*, Washington, DC: Davis & Force.

Nebelkopf, E. and Phillips, M. (eds) (2004) *Healing and Mental Health for Native Americans: Speaking in Red*, New York: Altamira Press.

Norris, T., Vines, P. L., and Hoeffel, E. (2012) *The American Indian and Alaska Native Population: 2010* (2010 Census Briefs, Rep.), Washington, DC: US Census Bureau.

Passell, J. S. (1996) "The growing American Indian population, 1960–1990: Beyond demography," in Sandefur, G., Rindfuss, R., and Cohen, B. (eds) *Changing Numbers, Changing Needs: American Indian Demography and Public Health*, Washington, DC: National Academy Press.

Rhoades, E. (ed.) (2000) *American Indian Health: Innovations in Healthcare, Promotion, and Policy*, London: Johns Hopkins University Press.

Riverside San Bernardino County Indian Health (n.d.) Available online at: www. rsbcihi.org (accessed October 29, 2008).

Schoolcraft, H. R. (1857) *History of the Indian Tribes of the United States: Their Present Condition and Prospects, and a Sketch of their Ancient Status*, Philadelphia, PA: J. B. Lippincott.

Snipp, C. M. (2000) "Selected demographic characteristics of Indians," in Rhoades, E. (ed.) *American Indian Health: Innovations in Healthcare, Promotion, and Policy*, London: Johns Hopkins University Press.

Spector, R. (2000) *Cultural Diversity in Health and Illness*, Upper Saddle River, NJ: Prentice Hall Health.

Sutton, C. and Nose, M. (2005) "American Indian families," in McGoldrick, M., Giordano, J., and Garcia-Preto, N. (eds) *Ethnicity & Family Therapy*, New York: The Guilford Press.

US Census Bureau (2000) *We the People: American Indians and Alaska Natives in the United States.* Available online at: www.census.gov/prod/2006pubs/censr-28.pdf (accessed September 28, 2016).

US Department of Health and Human Services: Indian Health Service (2015) *HIS Fact Sheet.* Available online at: www.ihs.gov/newsroom/factsheets/ihsyear-2015profile/ (accessed June 13, 2016).

Yale Law School, Lillian Goldman Law Library (n.d.) *Treaty with the Delawares: 1778.* Available online at: http://avalon.law.yale.edu/18th_century/del1778.asp (accessed October 20, 2008).

Suggested texts

Duran, E. (2006) *Healing the Soul Wound: Counseling with American Indians and other Native Peoples*, New York: Teachers College Press.

Fixico, D. (2003) *The American Indian Mind in a Linear World*, New York: Routledge.

Rhoades, E. M. D. (ed.) (2000) *American Indian Health: Innovations in Healthcare, Promotion, and Policy*, London: Johns Hopkins University Press.

Trafzer, C. and Weiner, D. (eds) (2001) *Medicine Ways: Disease, Health, and Survival among Native Americans*, New York: Altamira Press.

Witko, T. (ed.) (2006) *Mental Healthcare for Urban Indians*, Washington, DC: American Psychological Association.

4 Hinduism

Manoj Shah and Siroj Sorajjakool

Fear not what is not real, never was and never will be.
What is real, always was and cannot be destroyed.

Bhagavat Gita

Introduction

Hinduism, the third largest religion in the world, represents a collection of beliefs, practices, and ethos that arose in India around 1500 BCE. It is rooted in the *Vedas* and the history of the people of India and connected by *sanatana dharma*, "eternal duty," which suggests a common orientation toward liberation from the cycle of birth and rebirth (Young 2005: 58–9).

The term Hinduism is in itself complex and requires careful analysis so as to represent it more accurately. The religion that we now call Hinduism has "no historical founder, no single scriptural text recognized by all, no single authoritative voice or organization or institution, no common creed" (Schmidt et al. 1999: 208). While the history of Hinduism may be traced back to 1500 BCE, the designation "Hindu" was used much later and referred to the people of the Indus Valley. This new designation came as an attempt to create a religious distinction when Islam came to India.

Another complication with the term Hinduism is the diversity of beliefs and practices found within the religion. There are many gods with various ritual beliefs and practices. Despite these many variations of beliefs and practices, the common thread that holds things together appears to be the social traditions of those who follow Hinduism. Prakash Desai, professor of clinical psychiatry at the University of Illinois, explains:

Perhaps here lies the secret of the survival of the Hindu tradition. Accumulating various interpretations of reality, Hindus arrive at a vision of the good life determined by adaptation and accommodation to prevailing conditions. As the subcultures of multiple ethnic groups were being assimilated into a social order, regulation of behavior appears to have been more important than regulation of beliefs. The private lives of the populace were left alone, and in early India few attempts were made at consolidating a social philosophy that would then govern both public and private behavior. The result is a profound conviction that "truth" or self-realization is discovered through many paths, and a simultaneous rejection of absolutes in consideration of personal morality.

(Desai 1989: 11)

Hence the diversity of beliefs and practices are closely connected to the social traditions of the people of the Indus Valley creating unity within these variations, which is now called Hinduism.

Demographics

There are approximately one billion Hindus in the world, comprising 15 percent of the world population. This makes Hinduism the third largest religion in the world (Liu 2012). As of 2011, 79.8 percent of the population in India belongs to the Hindu religious faith (Census Organization of India 2011). The other major countries in which Hindus reside are Nepal, Bangladesh, Indonesia (especially Bali), Sri Lanka, Pakistan, Indonesia, and other Southeast Asian countries such as Malaysia, Singapore, and Thailand. According to a survey conducted by the Graduate Center of the City University of New York in 2001, there are 766,000 Hindus living in the United States, comprising 0.4 percent of the total population (Kosmin et al. 2001: 13). More recently, in 2014, the Pew Research Center recorded that this population is now 0.7 percent of the population (Pew Research Center 2015).

History

The foundation of Hinduism can be traced back to ancient, anonymous Indian sages who claimed to discover the eternal truths. These truths are called *apaurusheya* (not of human invention) as sages realized that these truths had always existed and had come from God (Bhaskarananda 2002: 4). These sages were called *rishis* (seers) because they had seen or experienced these truths with their purified minds. Hinduism is always evolving, thanks to various sages and saints who have enriched this religion with their teachings. The eternal truths were compiled by sage Vyasa in a book called the *Vedas*. Since then, many different saints, Adi Sankaracharya, Vallabhacharya, and Swami Vivekananda, to name a few, have reformed and revitalized Hinduism and made it relevant to their times. These flexible and evolving characteristics have prompted scholars to describe Hinduism as a way of life rather than a religion.

By the second millennium BCE there was a highly developed civilization in the northwestern part of the south Asian subcontinent called the Indus Valley, which is now a part of Pakistan. Archeologists have discovered two sites that indicate a high level of social order and planning. These sites are

Mohenjo-Daro and Harappa and they once formed a part of a larger social network (Schmidt et al. 1999: 222). By 1500 BCE, a semi-nomadic group called the Aryans invaded this region. The origin of the Aryans is a topic of controversy among scholars. It has been postulated that they may have come from Central Asia (Gafurov 1973: 141, 149), Lithuania (Bender 1922: 55), the Arctic (Tilak 1956: 388–9), or southeastern Europe (Bongard 1980: 123). Recently, it has been suggested that Indian Aryans were indigenous to India (Vivekananda 1947: 293). The Aryans brought with them their gods and their hierarchical social class. The religious rites of purification and the class system were used to preserve and elevate their race and subjugate the Dravidians, the aboriginals.

The history of religious development in Hinduism is rather complex due to various contributing factors such as the rise of Buddhism, Jainism, Islam, Christianity, and other socio-political developments. Hence it is difficult to place an exact time frame (Radhakrishnan 1956: vol. 2, 22–3). However, the religious development dating back to the arrival of the Aryans in the Indus Valley may be broadly divided into four main periods: the Vedic period (2000–600 BCE), the Ancient period (600 BCE–1000 CE), the Medieval period (1000–1800 CE), and the Modern period (1800–present) (Radhakrishnan 1956: vol. 1, 272).

The Vedic period (2000–600 BCE) represents the earliest developments of the Hindu religion and shows significant theological progression in the understanding of reality and cosmology. There were four major religious and theological texts that this period produced, referred to as *Samhitas*, *Brahmanas*, *Aranyakas*, and *Upanishads*.

Samhitas refers to the collection of ancient sayings and consists of four collections of the *Vedas*. The *Rig-Veda* is the earliest *Veda*, dealing with higher gods as conceived by a more advanced class. The *Sama-Veda* is the book of chants. *Yajur-Veda* contains liturgy (including mantras) essential for sacrifices in the religious practice during the Vedic period. Finally, *Atharva-Veda* represents a much more primitive stage of thought in comparison to other *Vedas*.

The cosmology of this era consisted of the personification of the gods in relation to their historical contexts. There were Mitra, the god of light; Surya, the sun god; Savitr, the god of the solar system; Agni, the god of fire; Soma, the god of breath and inspiration; Varuna, the god of the sky; and Indra, the god of thunder. Gradually, depending on their environmental and historical context, one of the gods became the preferred deity, though other gods were not rejected (henotheism). Indra was essential in matters of war, and Varuna for their agricultural concerns. Varuna was soon given the task of maintaining justice and morality. His role was to watch over the world, punish evil doers, and forgive those who ask for forgiveness. Gradually the concept of *rta* was developed. *Rta* refers to the cosmic order of the universe and the law of righteousness. Varuna, therefore, was the one who implemented the laws of *rta*.

Brahmanas are commentaries on the four *Vedas*, detailing the proper performance of rituals. The *Brahmanas* were seminal in the development of later Hindu thought and scholarship. During the *Samhitas* period, the movement grew from polytheism to henotheism. The *Brahmanas* helped move the developing Hinduism from henotheism to monotheism and from monotheism to monism. The crowding of the gods and goddesses proved to be exhausting to the intellect that seeks pattern and unity. Factors leading to the development of monotheism during this period were the belief in one and only one Supreme Being, unity in this world, and the idea of *rta*. Through these three factors there emerged the understanding of one supreme God. This supreme God was called Visvakarma (maker of the world), sometimes also Prajapati (lord of creatures).

Aranyakas provided the continuity from the *Brahmanas* in the sense that they dealt with the meanings of the "secret" rituals not detailed in the *Brahmanas*. The *Aranyakas* discuss dangerous sacrifices in the style of the *Brahmanas* and thus are primarily concerned with the proper performance of ritual. The *Aranyakas* are "secret" in the sense that they are restricted to a particular class of rituals that were conveyed individually from the teacher to the student.

Still the Hindu mind was not satisfied with deities that embodied human projections. Even the belief in the Supreme Being could not satisfy the search for a unifying principle and the essence of things. This led to the belief that there must be an impersonal ruling force in the universe. "There was then neither non-entity nor entity.... That One breathed calmly, self-supported; then was nothing different from it, or above it" (Muir 1967: 357). This theological development prepared the stage for the next significant religious period, the *Upanishads*.

Upanishads represents one of the most significant religious and philosophical developments during the Vedic period. The term *Upanishads* means to sit nearby or to be mentored by the learned, the sage. *Upanishads*, also called *Vedanta* (the height or culmination of knowledge), represented a very philosophical understanding of life and reality. It aimed at searching for a release from pain and suffering and claimed that attachment to that which is impermanent results in suffering. To escape from suffering, one needs to be attached to that which is permanent. That which is permanent is real. What is that which is permanent? According to *Upanishads*, at the essential core of each of us there is the absolute, constant, permanent, and unchanging bliss called *atman*. And this absolute bliss in each of us is of the same essence as Brahman. Hence the *Upanishads* teaches that *atman* is Brahman. Nothing else is real except Brahman and our attachment to the phenomenal world of change as a result of our ignorance is the primary cause of suffering. According to the *Upanishads*:

> Smaller than the smallest, greater than the greatest, this Self forever dwells within the hearts of all. When a man is free from desire, his

mind and senses purified, he beholds the glory of the Self and is
without sorrow.

(Prabhavananda and Manchester 1957: 123–4)

The Ancient Period (600 BCE–1000 CE) was an era of myths and narratives
and the development of six philosophical systems leading to a more refined
approach to *Vedanta* (the union between self and Brahman). The myths
and narratives were produced to convey spiritual teachings and lessons.
These narratives emerged as a response to challenges by Jainism and Buddhism on the Brahmanic teachings, rituals, and the caste system. A new
form of religious literature was needed to provide teachings that could
address the masses in a meaningful way. Chief among the stories of this
period were the two great Indian epics, *Ramayana* and *Mahabarata*.
Ramayana tells the story of Rama (the divine incarnation of Vishnu, the
god of preservation), who abides by the law of *dharma*, the prescription
for ways of conducting oneself within the religious and social realms.
Rama portrayed the qualities of an obedient son, a faithful husband, and a
responsible ruler. However, because his stepmother wished for her own
son to become the ruler of Aydohya instead of Rama, he was banished to
the forest for fourteen years. His faithful wife, Sita, and his brother, Lak-
shmana, joined him in the forest. While in the forest, the evil king of
Lanka, Ravana, abducted Sita. Rama solicited the help of the monkey king
Hanuman, built a bridge to Lanka, and brought Sita safely back to
Aydohya. Once they returned to Aydohya, Rama demanded under the
pressure of the public that Sita prove her purity before he could receive her
back. She did so by walking over a large fire without harm. *Ramayana*
describes the ideal way of life exemplified by different characters in the
epic, showing the importance of living life according to *dharma*.

 Mahabarata tells the story of the conflict and war within a family and
the price of abiding by the *dharma*. Within *Mahabarata* is a section called
Bhagavat Gita (The Song of the Lord), which is one of the most influential
sacred texts in Hinduism. In *Bhagavat Gita*, Prince Arjuna of the Pandavas
family expresses his anxiety regarding going to battle against his own
cousins during a civil war. Lord Krishna, the incarnation of Vishnu, serves
as the king's charioteer and while riding into battle taught Arjuna an
important lesson on *dharma*. The *Bhagavat Gita* contains 700 verses of
dialogue between Krishna and Arjuna regarding the detachment of oneself
from the consequence of one's own actions. *Dharma* calls us to act rightly
and be willing to accept whatever consequences may come. It is not our
duty to attach ourselves to the consequences of our action whether that be
positive or negative. We are called to act in accord with *dharma* and that
is our sole responsibility. In *Bhagavat Gita*, Lord Krishna instructs Arjuna:

 There are principles to regulate attachment and aversion pertaining to
 the senses and their objects. One should not come under the control of

such attachment and aversion, because they are stumbling blocks on the path of self-realization. It is far better to discharge one's prescribed duties, even though faultily, than another's duties perfectly. Destruction in the course of performing one's own duty is better than engaging in another's duties, for to follow another's path is dangerous.

(Prabhupada 1997: 116–17)

There was also the development of six philosophical systems (*darshanas*) aiming at offering intellectual defense against challenges posted by Jainism and Buddhism. The authors of the six systems wrote treatises using very concise aphorisms called sutras. The first two are *Nyaya* and *Vaisheshika*, which are collections of sutras that provide logic and cosmology, while *Samkhya* offers the basis for the teachings of *Bhagavat Gita*. *Yoga* teaches the discipline of the body as a method of achieving detachment, and *Mimamsa* explores rituals. Finally, *Vedanta* discusses the relationship between the self and Brahman. Within *Vedanta*, there are three major approaches. In *Advaita*, as popularized by Shankara, there is ultimately no distinction between the self and Brahman. *Dvaita* of Ramanuja suggests that there is a radical difference between the self and Brahman while *Dvaitadvaita* leaves room for possible tension between these two possibilities (Schmidt et al. 1999: 232–3).

Hindu religious practices during the medieval period (1000–1800 CE) placed emphasis on the place of *bhakti* (devotion). *Bhakti* refers to the belief that liberation can be achieved through total devotion through singing and chanting often associated with strong emotion and mystical experience with the deity, the type of relationship that is comparable to that between the lover and the beloved (Britannica 2008). Bhakti as a movement originated from South India and the two main deities were Vishnu (the god who preserves) and Shiva (the god who destroys and recreates). Those who worship Vishnu are called Vaishanavaite and those who worship Shiva are called Shaivite (Hawkins 2004: 49–64).

The modern period (1800–present) in the development of Hinduism in many ways emerged from an attempt to respond to the influence of Christianity and Western thought. An important development during this era is the religious movement called Brahmo Samaj, founded by Ram Mohan Roy (1772–1833). It was the movement that focused on eliminating discrimination against women, especially that of *sati* (burning of widows along with their deceased husbands), incorporating certain aspects of Christianity, and promoting English-style schools for children. Rabindranath Tagore (the first Indian Nobel laureate) continued the work of Brahmo Samaj and established a Bengali language newspaper and a school for Brahmo Samaj missionaries. Another significant movement during this period came from a Brahmin priest of the Kali temple in Calcutta. Ramakrishna (1836–1886), who attracted many followers in Calcutta, preached the message of unity of all religions and invited many to renounce worldly possessions and become monks. The teachings of Ramakrishna came to Europe and America through the influential work of one of his followers, Vivekananda (1863–1902), founder of Ramakrishna Mission. He is credited as a major figure in the revival of Hinduism in India (Hawkins 2004: 91–4).

Beliefs and practices

General

The practices of Hinduism are based on the beliefs and teachings of the *Vedas*. According to the *Vedas*, there is one Supreme God called Brahman. Other terms used to describe this transcendental God are Absolute Truth, Consciousness, Infinite Bliss, Impersonal God, and Nirguna (attribute-less) Brahman. However, it is very difficult to think of the infinite Brahman with one's finite mind. Thus, the idea of Nirguna Brahman gave way to Saguna Brahman, or Personal God. This Personal God, also known as Ishvara, has three basic aspects: (1) the creator called Brahma, (2) the preserver called Vishnu, and (3) the destroyer called Shiva. There are many other aspects of this Personal God, and each of these other aspects can be personified as a deity. The deities are not so much different gods; they are the personifications of various aspects of one and the same Ishvara. For example, when Hindus pray for knowledge or learning, they think of Ishvara personified as deity Saraswati (goddess of knowledge). This results in the common misunderstanding that there are many gods in Hinduism. Ultimately, Hinduism asserts one Supreme God and the goal of believers is to merge with this God.

The *Vedas* speaks of the law of eternal duty, or *sanatana dharma*, and refers to the cycle of birth and rebirth (*samsara*) resulting in pain and suffering due to bad deeds (*karma*) and in the path of liberation (*moksha*). These three concepts form the basis for Hindu beliefs and practices. According to the *Vedas*, one's true nature is that of eternal, unchanging self or *atman*. It is to be differentiated from the material and changing self. But through ignorance of the true nature of self, we become attached to this false, physical self, thereby causing a karmic reaction.

The word karma comes from the root *kri*, which means "to do." Every action becomes karma. These actions are judged and evaluated by the law of causation that states, "You reap what you sow." The concept of karma, derived from *rta*, first appeared in the *Vedas*. *Rta* was the principle that governed both physical and moral actions. During the *Brahmanas* period, it was looked upon as a fixed law of causation applying to all moral conduct. According to this law, every act carries with it an effect. This law does not only apply to this life but extends to the next life as well, associating the doctrine of karma to the doctrine of reincarnation (the cycle of birth and rebirth). The law does not only judge one's external behavior, but also one's intentions behind any given action.

But if a person's life is in accordance with the law of karma, is this person's life pre-determined? Where is the place of freedom? The tension of karma and freedom may be explained on the basis of the three forms of karma. First, *prarabdha* karma may be compared to an arrow that has already been discharged. It refers to fully pre-determined things such as gender, parents, and the color of one's skin. This type of karma is responsible for the pleasures and pains of this present life. Second, *samchita* karma is like an arrow resting in the bow about to be discharged and refers primarily to character and innate tendencies. It is still possible, in this view of karma, to change one's character and overcome one's tendencies. This change can be achieved by ritualistic acts and through *jnana* (knowledge). *Samchita* karma is accumulated over many past lives and results in good things in future lives. Third, *agami* karma is the arrow that has not yet been placed in the bow. This refers to any action that is performed in this life and may affect results in both this life and the next. *Agami* karma that does not bear any results in this life becomes accumulated as *samchita* karma. Through these various forms of karma, each one of us is the creator and architect of our future. We shape our own life and everything we do has natural consequences.

Samsara, or the cycle of birth and rebirth, is a natural development of the concept of karma. *Samsara* refers to the cycle of birth and rebirth that will continue unceasing as long as karma exists. Karma and *samsara* also help explain the problem of suffering. As long as one is engaged in negative mental, emotional, and behavioral processes, one will remain within this cycle of pain and suffering. The source of rebirth includes the fear of death, the love for the deceased, the illusion regarding the reality of life, and the desire to live. The way out of this suffering is through *moksha*.

The term *moksha* means liberation or emancipation from selfishness, ignorance, and attachment. It is the path that releases one from the cycle of birth and rebirth that causes suffering. The four paths leading to *moksha* are:

1   *Jnana marga* (the path of knowledge). This is the path of liberation through the attainment of right knowledge and understanding. If we do not understand the cause of suffering it would be impossible to be released from *samsara*.
2   *Karma marga* (the path of action). This is the path of liberation through right action, through good deeds that include the correct performance of ritual and sacrifices.
3   *Raj yoga marga* (the path of discipline). The practice of yoga through the discipline of the body and mind can enhance one's concentration on divinity and results in the reduction of bad karma.
4   *Bhakti marga* (the path of devotion). Through devotion of total and fully committed love for God one may achieve liberation.

While life's ultimate goal is to achieve *moksha*, Hindus recognize the importance of various stages of life that one must go through as one matures. First, it is important to practice *dharma*, or good moral conduct, because morality occupies the highest place in Hindu thought. Second, *artha*, or wealth, is an important part of life. A person must work hard to sustain and provide for the family. It is important to remember that earning must be done in an honest manner. The third stage refers to *kama*, worldly desire or pleasure. To acknowledge the realm of passion is to acknowledge the reality of human nature. In Hindu tradition there is nothing wrong with worldly desire as long as it is expressed in appropriate ways. Finally, there is *moksha*. In this final stage the goal is to arrive at *sanyasin*, to be "one who neither hates nor loves anything." This is the stage where one no longer yearns to be "somebody." A *sanyasin* is contented with life and finds harmony within the self. It may be contrasted with the unwise life where one struggles with aging, life, and death.

Health and disease

Health beliefs and practices among Hindus may be dated back to 5000 BCE when sages searched for solutions to the problem of ill health and disease. During the early stage of development, disease was viewed as a punishment from the gods or perturbation of the demons. When transgression took place the god Varuna, who governed moral law, was understood to cause diseases as punishment, while Rudra, the god of ambivalence, inflicted pain at random. According to A. L. Basham, "Demons as causes of disease loom large in the later collection of hymns known as the Atharva Veda," pointing to the general belief "that illness was caused by evil spirits, who could be expelled by the utterance of the right formula by qualified practitioners, often aided by the administration of herbal remedies and other treatments" (Basham 1998: 19). However, by the sixth or fifth century BCE, the Indian medical system had evolved into its current form. This medical evolution has come to be known as *Ayurveda*, the science of life and longevity about which most Indians possess basic understanding. Ayurvedic medicine is divided into eight categories: (1) general principles of medicine, (2) pathology, (3) diagnosis, (4) physiology and anatomy, (5) prognosis, (6) therapeutics, (7) pharmaceutics, and (8) treatment protocol (Basham 1998: 20). But *Ayurveda* is "not merely a system of medicine"; rather it is "a way of life that aims to increase lifespan by preventing or delaying the aging process. Its objective is to create optimal health and well-being through a comprehensive approach that addresses mind, body, behavior, and environment" (Sharma et al. 2007: 1012).

In Ayurvedic terms, health is the balance between body, mind, and spirit. It is about diet and exercise. It consists of the way we see the world. It speaks of the quality of our souls. It believes in positive social relation and perspective in life. It is the perspective that helps reduce stress and encourages balanced living, the type of living that takes time to love, laugh, eat, play, work, and relate to other human beings in a meaningful way.

From the perspective of wholeness and balance, the human body consists of three basic elements. These are wind (*vata*), fire (*pitta*), and water (*kapha*). A healthy body results from harmonic balance of these three elements. When any of its elements are out of balance, the system becomes "troubled" (Obeyesekere 1998: 201–2). Desai explains that "an excess of *fire* will produce fever, redness, burning, smells, and discoloration; an excess of *wind* will produce paralysis, cramps, fainting, deafness, and joint pains; and the symptoms of aggravated *moisture* are drowsiness, lethargy, swelling, and stiffness" (Desai 1989: 82). There are two things that may cause imbalance in a person. There are the external factors such as pollution, changing seasons, and infection, and the internal factors such as stress, internal conflicts, and grief. When the internal is toxic, it weakens the body and hence decreases its ability to fight or resist harmful external factors. The causes for internal toxins are fear, anxiety, anger, greed, sorrow, and envy. The fire element may be aggravated by passion and anger. Sorrow and grief can trouble the moisture, while vanity negatively impacts the wind element (Desai 1989: 82). The build-up of internal toxins can be explained by understanding how blockage within the internal system affects the body. Poor blood circulation resulting from blockage has a negative impact on the distribution of nutrition, reduces the flow of oxygen, and results in various physical symptoms such as fatigue, dizziness, and heart palpitation. A journalist, Shubhra Krishan, who spent many years studying Ayurvedic medicine, describes this process:

> On a rushed day, I go on my toxin-collecting spree more systematically. I work late into the night, depriving my body and mind of the rest they need. I wake up irritable and groggy, with little appetite for breakfast. Whatever appetite I have, I douse with three continuous cups of coffee. I go to work and plunge straightaway into the waiting files. I make careless mistakes, then simmer when they're pointed out. Just before a crucial meeting, I find I have gone completely blank. How do these acts of neglect translate into actual toxins? They generate such substance as acid, bile, cholesterol, and adrenaline. In moderate amounts, these are essential to life. But produced in excess, they overwhelm the body, compromising its ability to perform the routine functions of metabolism and digestion normally.
>
> (Krishan 2003: 19–20)

In Ayurvedic terms, these toxins are called *ama*, which means "unripe, immature, undigested" (Krishan 2003: 20). Before we can understand the Ayurvedic approach to cleansing toxins from the body it is important to understand the concept of personal constitution. Each person comes with a core constitution and the constitution emerges from the combination of five basic elements: earth, water, wind, fire, and ether. Because every human being is a microcosm of the universe, these elements are present in each individual. The basic nature of each individual may be divided into three categories: *vata* (ether and air), *pitta* (earth and fire), and *kapha* (water and earth), resulting from various possible combinations of the five elements. Understanding these basic types can help us understand how to restore health and balance.

An individual leaning toward *vata* (wind) tends to be quick in thought and action, and light and thin in build, has dry skin, is sensitive to cold, a light sleeper, tends to worry, and responds positively to warm, cooked foods and hot beverages. A *pitta* (fire) person has a moderate build, strong appetite and digestion, reddish complexion, is sensitive to hot weather, has a steady memory, can be irritable and is quick-tempered, a perfectionistic and responds well to cold food and beverages. A *kapha* (water) person is normally heavy in build, has great endurance, is slow and methodical, has oily skin, a calm and steady personality, is a heavy sleeper, has slow digestion and mild appetite, and has thick and dark hair (Krishan 2003: 49–51).

Harmonic balance and imbalance may differ from type to type. Factors that cause imbalance in *vata* are: bitter, salty, and astringent tastes, dryness, light, cold foods, late night sleep, excessive exercise, grief, and worry. For *pitta*, imbalance may be caused by pungent, sour, and salty tastes, heat exposure, exhaustion, and anger. *Kapha* persons become imbalanced through sweet, sour, and salty tastes, oily and heavy foods, overeating, lack of exercise, excess sleeping, or napping. Further there are factors that can cause imbalance for all types. These are: eating excessively, improper diet, contaminated food, foul and dry meat, eating food out of season, negative thoughts, and being inactive (Tirtha 1998: 40–1). *Ayurveda* recognizes that different foods, tastes, climates, colors, seasons, and activities affect people differently depending on their basic types. Hence when one recognizes one's type and learns to observe one's responses to diet, environment, seasons, and psychological factors, one may learn to achieve and maintain balance within oneself and thus achieve good health.

As part of the attempt to balance the health system, *Ayurveda* recommends a cleansing process called *panchakarma* (five actions) to get rid of toxins from the body. As the name indicates, this process involves five procedures as follows: (1) vomiting, (2) purgation, (3) enema, (4) elimination of toxins through the nose, and (5) moksha, detoxification of blood.

Hindus approach various health and bioethical issues with a deep reverence for scripture and tradition, though not without sensitivity to modern medicine and technology. On birth control, the *Vedas* do not make a specific prohibition against it, and many modern Hindus practice some form of birth control. As far as abortion is concerned, Hindu scriptures such as the *Rig-Veda, Atharva Veda*, and *Sushruta Samhita* prohibit abortion, except when the mother's life is in danger. This is primarily because Hinduism is a religion of non-violence. Furthermore, because of the Hindu belief in reincarnation, abortion may be viewed as a negative process that interferes with the cycle of life in accord with one's karma, especially since most Hindus believe that the soul exists at conception. However, attitudes toward elective termination of pregnancy vary among modern Hindus (Coward and Sidhu 2000: 1167–70; Jootum 2002: 38–40; Coward 2004: 2759–60).

When considering the issue of diet, most Hindus are lacto-vegetarians and avoid animal products, except milk, in the diet. Even among those who consume animal products, beef and pork are strongly avoided. It is important when working with patients to explain the source of medications, like insulin or pancreatic enzymes, whether or not they come from animal sources. Also, there are certain days of the month and year when fasting is observed in accord with special occasions, mostly related to their personal deities. Fasting is considered to be purifying.

Another issue that needs to be taken into consideration is that of biotechnology. Advances in biotechnology and medical treatments such as stem cell research have further complicated Hindus' approach to healthcare and ethics. There are no historical examples of such innovations in scripture, making present-day recommendations difficult. However, there are various governmental agencies in India, such as the Department of Biotechnology and the Indian Council of Medical Research, who help provide answers to the moral and ethical questions arising from the use of biotechnology (Jayaraman 1997: 838; Mudur 2001: 530).

Death and dying

Hindus believe the body is a vehicle for the soul or *atman* through which it can experience the world and progress on its journey to God. At the time of death, this body is discarded and *atman* takes on another body; this cycle of changing bodies continues until *atman* reaches its final goal – union with God. Hindus believe that *atman* is immortal, while the physical body is perishable. They believe that suffering at the time of death is due to *karma* and therefore inevitable. Many prefer to die at home and may want to have specific ritual or religious rites performed. Many prefer to listen to sacred chants from scriptures and have drops of sacred water from the Ganges River put in their mouth at the time of death. A dying person may wish to be moved to the floor to be close to Mother Earth. After death, close family members wash the body; a priest may perform religious rites; then the body is cremated, preferably within twenty-four hours. Children younger than three years of age are usually simply buried, however. There is a ten to fourteen day period of family mourning. Since death is seen as a period of transition into the next life, excessive mourning is discouraged. During this period of mourning, family members do not perform religious ceremonies. They eat simple vegetarian food and wear white clothing as a symbol of mourning. At the end of the mourning period, a religious ceremony is performed to ensure that the deceased has a peaceful transition to the next life.

Suicide is perceived as a bad way to die and a reprehensible act. Similarly, euthanasia is discouraged. Artificial life support is not viewed favorably as most Hindus believe that prolonging life after a person's time for death interferes with *karma* and disrupts the cycle of reincarnation. Organ donation and transplants are acceptable and not subject to the same laws on non-violence, since the donors chose to give of themselves out of their own free will (unlike animals). Some Hindus, however, disagree as they believe every action has karmic implications and something as serious as replacing a major organ can carry some of the donor's *karma* to the recipient. Additionally, some believe that since a part of the deceased donor's physical body still "lives" this may interfere with the donor's soul moving on to the next incarnation.

Conclusion

Hinduism is a complex religion that accommodates a wide variation in beliefs and practices in relation to conceptual understanding of deities and related rituals and rites. However, within these wide variations we find

Table 4.1 Dos and don'ts

Dos	Don'ts
1 Be aware of philosophical reasons for particular behaviors or decisions in medical care.	1 Do not remove jewelry, adornments, or threads without discussing with patient as they have religious significance.
2 Recognize that fasting is a common practice and may affect medical/ dietary plans.	2 Do not disregard family members when making medical decisions.
3 Be sensitive to concerns about modesty.	3 Do not use left hand (if possible) when performing tasks on the patients (due to cultural understanding of cleanliness) and be cautious when handling patient's hand movement in any way (starting an intravenous line etc.).
4 Discuss possibility of imminent death with family members regarding location or religious rituals and rites.	
5 Provide same-sex caregivers.	
6 Understand that strong belief in astrology may prevent a family from naming a newborn before leaving the hospital or agreeing to a certain time for elective surgery.	4 Do not disregard times for prayer or meditation and avoid medical procedures or examinations during those times.
7 Understand that pain and suffering may be seen as the result of *karma* and may impact the patient's self-report of pain.	5 Do not disregard dietary preference and patients' hesitation to use medications with animal by-products.
8 Take into account ideas about "hot" and "cold" food theory in Ayurvedic thought.	6 Do not touch Hindu scriptures with feet or put them on the floor as to do so would be a grave insult.
9 Remove shoes before entering the Hindu home (home healthcare workers).	
10 Note the exact time of birth.	

common themes permeating the world of Hindu religious beliefs – the path leading to oneness with Brahman, the Ultimate Reality, as a symbol of eternal bliss, and the practice of non-violence toward life. In relation to health, religion plays a significant role in showing the connection between physical wellbeing and Hindu cosmology. By pursuing optimal health through the balance between the body, the mind, and the spirit, Hindus seek to experience wholeness in this life and build positive karma for the lives to come – until they ultimately reach *moksha*.

Case study

Used simply, the word "karma" in the United States is widely used, even if usually misunderstood. Though there are many synonyms for the word, its most common sense of use regards the idea that "what goes around comes around." In other words, the actions we may engage in today will have results sometime in the future that we cannot predict today. The religious use of *karma* in Hinduism, however, is vastly more complicated. Recently, I ran into the use of this word that resulted in my insulting a case worker at the hospital.

We were discussing a case in which the patient was being discharged back home under the care of a local hospice. She was the social worker active on her case and was telling me about how difficult the discharge had been. In her view, the family had been very hard to work with. They all seemed comfortable with their matriarch going home in the full knowledge that she would likely die soon from her cancer. But something had got in the way according to her. She worked for the palliative care service at the hospital. The patient's care had been well managed by the palliative care team and it did not appear there were any problems with moving back home and taking up with the local hospice. The patient and her family were clearly Hindu and I had already worked with our spiritual care department to make sure that our Chaplain, who was most well informed and connected in the Hindu community, was working with them. The case worker, however, was not tuned in to the religious realities of the patient and her family.

The case worker and I were reviewing the case because the hospital patient experience department had received a complaint about her work. According to the family, something had gone wrong during one of her conversations so we were going over it in very close detail. I had asked her what religion the family was and she replied that she was not sure but did not think they were Christian. In describing her conversation with me, she said at one point, "I told them that I thought they might want to consider the State's new Assisted Suicide law, but that karma on that sort of thing might be a bitch." I paused slightly before asking her in response, "What is karma?" She said something about destiny and reincarnation, so I asked again, "What is karma?" Looking a bit confused, but working with me, she said, "Well, it's when you do something wrong, eventually something wrong will happen to you." So, I changed my question ever so slightly, "Where does the word 'karma' come from?" Now clearly upset, she responded that she did not know, but that it had something to do with reincarnation.

Questions for reflection

1 Do licensed clinical social workers have any responsibility to know anything about Hinduism?
2 Can we fault someone growing up in America these days for using common vernacular that has come to us from particular religious traditions through the process of immigration?
3 Is the family really the problem here? Could they/should they have simply described the importance of karma in their life and thought about death and reincarnation?

Glossary

Atman   The true self that transcends the phenomenal world of our daily existence.

Ayurveda   This term means the science of life and refers to the system of traditional medicine native to India.

Bhagavat Gita   One of the sacred scriptures in Hinduism containing 700 verses of conversation between Krishna and Arjuna regarding the path toward self-realization. It also forms a part of the larger text, the *Mahabarata*.

Brahman   The Divine ground of all reality that is unchanging, infinite, unconditional, and immanent.

Dharma   The path leading to righteous living.

Karma   An action or deed governed by the law of causality that can result in positive or negative direction in future lives and in the cycle of birth and rebirth.

Moksha   This equates with salvation, the final liberation from the cycle of birth and rebirth, resulting in union with Brahman.

Samsara   The cycle of birth and rebirth.

Vedas   The term Vedas means "knowledge" and refers to the oldest compilation of sacred scriptures in the Hindu tradition.

Bibliography

Basham, A. L. (1998) "The practice of medicine in ancient and medieval India," in Leslie, C. (ed.) *Asian Medical Systems: A Comparative Study*, Berkeley, CA: University of California Press.

Bender, H. H. (1922) *The Home of the Indo-Europeans*, New Jersey: Princeton University Press.

Bhaskarananda, S. (2002) *The Essentials of Hinduism: A Comprehensive Overview of the World's Oldest Religion*, Seattle, WA: Viveka Press.

Bongard, G. M. (1980) *The Origin of the Aryans*, Delhi, India: Arnold-Heinemann.

Britannica (2008) "Bhakti," in *Encyclopædia Britannica*, Chicago, IL: Encyclopædia Britannica. Available online at: www.britannica.com/topic/bhakti (accessed September 29, 2016).

Census Organization of India (2011) *Religion Census 2011*. Available online at: www.census2011.co.in/religion.php (accessed June 16, 2016).

Coward, H. (2004) "Hindu bioethics for the twenty-first century," *Journal of the American Medical Association*, vol. 291, no. 22: 2759–60.

Coward, H. and Sidhu, T. (2000) "Bioethics for clinicians: Hinduism and Sikhism," *Canadian Medical Association Journal*, vol. 163, no. 9: 1167–70.

Desai, P. (1989) *Health and Medicine in the Hindu Tradition*, New York: Crossroad.

Gafurov, B. G. (1973) *From Ancient History to Contemporary Times Central Asia*, Delhi, India: Navyug.

Hawkins, B. (2004) *Asian Religions*, New York: Pearson/Longman.

Jayaraman, K. S. (1997) "India may set up genetics advisory panel," *Nature*, vol. 387: 838.

Jootum, D. (2002) "Nursing with dignity – Part 7: Hinduism," *Nursing Times*, vol. 98, no. 15: 38–40.

Kosmin, B. A., Mayer, E., and Keysar, A. (2001) "American Religious Identification Survey 2001," *The Graduate Center of the City University of New York*. Available online at: www.gc.cuny.edu/CUNY_GC/media/CUNY-Graduate-Center/PDF/ARIS/ARIS-PDF-version.pdf (accessed September 29, 2016).

Krishan, S. (2003) *Essential Ayurveda: What It Is & What It Can Do for You*, Novato, CA: New World Library.

Liu, J. (2012) *Hindus*, Pew Research Center. Available online at: www.pewforum.org/2012/12/18/global-religious-landscape-hindu/ (accessed June 13, 2016).

Mudur, G. (2001) "India to tighten rules of human embryonic stem cell research," *British Medical Journal*, vol. 2001, no. 323: 530.

Muir, J. (1967) *Original Sanskrit Texts*, 2nd edn, Amsterdam: Oriental Press.

Obeyesekere, G. (1998) "The impact of Ayurvedic ideas on the culture and the individual in Sri Lanka," in Leslie, C. (ed.) *Asian Medical Systems: A Comparative Study*, Berkeley, CA: University of California Press.

Pew Research Center (2015) *America's Changing Religious Landscape*. Available online at: www.pewforum.org/2015/05/12/americas-changing-religious-landscape (accessed September 29, 2016).

Prabhavananda, S. and Manchester, F. (trans) (1957) *The Upanisads: Breath of the Eternal*, New York: Mentor Books.

Prabhupada, A. C. (1997) *Bhagavat-Gita As It Is*, Los Angeles: Bhaktivendata.

Radhakrishnan, S. (1956) *Indian Philosophy*, vols 1 and 2, Bombay: Blackie & Son.

Schmidt, R., Sager, G., Carney, G., Jackson, Jr., J., Muller, A., and Zanca, K. (1999) *Patterns of Religion*, Belmont, CA: Wadsworth Publishing.

Sharma, H., Chandola, H. M., Singh, G., and Basisht, G. (2007) "Utilization of Ayurveda in health care: An approach for prevention, health promotion, and treatment of disease; Part 1 – Ayurveda, the science of life," *The Journal of Alternative and Complementary Medicine*, vol. 13, no. 9: 1012.

Tilak, B. G. (1956) *The Arctic Home in Vedas*, Pune, India: Tilak Brothers.

Tirtha, S. S. (1998) *The Ayurveda Encyclopedia: Natural Secrets to Healing, Prevention, & Longevity*, Bayville, NY: Ayurveda Holistic Center Press.

Vivekananda, S. (1947) *The Complete Works of Swami Vivekanand*, vol. 3, Calcutta, India: Vedanta Press.

Young, W. (2005) *The World's Religions: Worldviews and Contemporary Issues*, New Jersey: Prentice Hall.

Suggested texts

Desai, P. (1989) *Health and Medicine in the Hindu Tradition*, New York: Crossroad.

Krishan, S. (2003) *Essential Ayurveda: What It Is & What It Can Do for You*, Novato, CA: New World Library.

Rodrigues, H. (2006) *Introducing Hinduism*, Oxford: Routledge.

Singhal, G. D. and Patterson, T. J. S. (1993) *Synopsis of Ayurveda: Based on a Translation of the Susruta Samhita* (The Treatise of Susruta), Oxford: Oxford University Press.

5 Buddhism

Siroj Sorajjakool and Supaporn Naewbood

As rain breaks through a poorly thatched house,
passion will break through an unreflecting mind.
As rain does not break through a well-thatched house,
passion will not break through a well-reflecting mind.
Dammapada

Introduction

Pain is often the reason that makes us ponder the deep meaning of life. It propels us toward this difficult quest until we discover the answer. But for a person to live in the presence of prosperity and comfort while determining to find the answer to this perplexing question, one has to be destined for this task. And this was the life of Gautama, the man who, although born into wealth and royalty, abandoned all in the quest for the solution to the question of suffering. Why suffering and what is the path that leads to the cessation of suffering?

Demographics

There are approximately 488 million Buddhists globally, which makes Buddhism the fourth largest religion (Liu 2012). The followers of Buddhism may be divided into three main schools of thought: Theravada Buddhism consists of 38 percent of the total Buddhist population (Nepal, India, Sri Lanka, Thailand, Myanmar, and Cambodia), 56 percent embraces Mahayana Buddhism (China, Japan, Korea, Taiwan, Vietnam, and Singapore), and 6 percent belongs to Tantric Buddhism (Tibet and parts of India) (Buddha Dharma Association and BuddhaNet n.d.). According to the National Survey of Religious Identification and the American Religious Identity Survey completed in 2008 regarding religious demographics in America, there are approximately 1.18 million Buddhists in the United States, which is approximately 0.5 percent of the total population (Kosmin and Keysar 2008: 7).

History

Siddharta Gautama was born around 565 BCE to the Shakya clan in Lumbini (which is now Nepal). His father was Suddhodana, the ruler of Kapilavastu, and his mother, Maya. The story is told that Maya had a night vision in which she saw a white elephant (symbolizing holiness) entering into her body. Nine months later she gave birth to Gautama in a garden in Lumbini. The day he was born, he walked seven steps and in the place where his footsteps fell lotus flowers blossomed. Seven days later his mother passed away. Not long after his birth, sage Asita announced to the king that this young prince would either become a great king or a great holy man. The sage's message persuaded Suddhodana to shield his son from any religious teachings and human tragedy. Under such a protective environment, Gautama grew up, married Yasodara, and had a son.

It seems, however, that nothing could prevent Gautama from the destiny to which he was called. Even in his comfortable life, he witnessed three human conditions that changed the entire course of his life. He saw sickness, old age, and death. And while pondering this human predicament, he came across an ascetic (someone exercising rigorous, severe self-discipline and self-denial). The image of this ascetic convinced him of his calling. In the middle of the night he left Yasodara and his son, Rahula. Discarding his robe and cutting his hair as a symbol of his decision to give up the life of abundance, he abandoned the palace in search for truth and liberation from pain and suffering.

For six years Gautama went through various forms of intense quest for liberation. He first attempted the Brahmanic meditative approach as taught in the Upanishads (Hindu sacred text). When that did not work, he committed himself to extreme asceticism where he wandered naked throughout the countryside, fasted continually, and often spent sleepless nights searching for truth. During this period five other ascetics joined him. Gautama realized that these ascetic practices only led to physical deterioration and not spiritual enlightenment. He came to the conclusion that both extremes (pleasure and self-denial) would not be beneficial spiritually and decided to take the middle path. In the region called Bodh Gaya, he sat under a bodhi tree and told himself that he would remain there until he discovered the truth about suffering and the path toward liberation. Sitting in a meditative position, Gautama was tempted by Mara, the Hindu god of desire, calling him to return to his life of pleasure and luxury. Firm in his commitment, Gautama continued his quest with his right hand pointing toward the earth (symbolizing the earth as his witness). While meditating under this bodhi tree he "awakened" from the slumber of worldly delusions and understood the cause and the way out of suffering. He became the enlightened Buddha. His emphasis on the "middle path" attracted many followers in India who were searching for liberation but found the esoteric teachings of the Upanishads difficult to achieve. He continued to proclaim his message and laid the foundation of the Buddhist order of monks for the next 45 years.

In 250 BCE a great division occurred among the leadership in Buddhism regarding enlightenment. Those who believed that enlightenment was for all called themselves Mahayana (the great vehicle), while the other group was known as Hinayana (the small vehicle). Because of the negative connotation, the Hinayana group began to call themselves Theravada (the Way of the Elders).

Theravada Buddhism is found mostly in India, Sri Lanka, Myanmar, Laos, Thailand, and Cambodia. According to Theravada Buddhism, the Buddha possessed many human qualities and was not insulated from making mistakes. The ethical teachings of Theravada Buddhism are to abstain from evil and the accumulation of material goods, purify one's mind through meditation, and gain right understanding through the Four Noble Truths. Philosophically, Theravada Buddhism emphasizes that nirvana is a state free from passion, ill will, and delusion. It is a state beyond description. An *arahat* is a person who arrives at this stage and therefore is able to end the cycle of birth and rebirth.

Mahayana Buddhism may be translated as "the big vessel" because it offers greater possibility for the attainment of liberation than in Theravada Buddhism. Mahayana Buddhism is commonly practiced in regions such as China, Japan, Taiwan, Korea, Singapore, and Vietnam. Among the more popular Mahayana schools are Zen, Pure Land, and Tantric Buddhism. Mahayana emphasizes meditation as an attempt to attain the state of quiescence. Its aim is to empty oneself and attain the transcendental state of mind. The Mahayana School believes that the Buddha is no longer the historical sage of the Sakyas clan but he is supra-mundane (above physical manifestation). Mahayana Buddhism teaches the concept of *Bodhicitta* or the awakening of consciousness emphasizing liberation through recognizing *sunyata* (emptiness) or the illusion of things that we are attached to resulting in entrapment within the cycle of pain and suffering. Through meditation one may be awakened and find liberation. The concept of *Boddhisatva* is also one of the main foci. This concept teaches that the goal of life is to be enlightened but that one must forgo entrance to nirvana in order to assist other creatures through compassion and wisdom, helping them discover the path for the cessation of suffering.

In India around 272 BCE King Ashoka's empire extended from southeast of the Caspian Sea to the Indus valley. At the end of the eight years of his reign, he invaded the country of Kalinga (Orissa), India. During this invasion many thousands died. Upon seeing the effect of war, King Ashoka was struck with sorrow and grief, which led him to embrace Buddhism and he adopted non-violence as the state policy. From his desire to spread this message, he sent representatives to Syria, Egypt, and Greece. His son Mahinda and his sister Samghamata went to Sri Lanka, which became a stronghold of Theravadins from that time on, while his other son, Kantana, took the message to the northwest of India. Theravada Buddhism continued to spread to Burma, Thailand, Cambodia, and Laos.

In China during the first century CE, Theravada Buddhism was introduced to China but the growth was slow. The emphasis on monasticism did not go well with the traditional concept of ancestor worship that promoted marriage and family. When Mahayana Buddhism was later introduced, the Chinese responded positively because the concept of heavenly beings in Mahayana could accommodate ancestor worship and sons who became Buddhists could continue to help their ancestors. Since that time, Mahayana Buddhism has continued to grow and spread to Japan, Tibet, Central Asia, Taiwan, Vietnam, and Korea (Matthews 1999: 149).

While it is believed that Buddhism was in conversation with the Western world as early as the first century CE, it became much more visible in the nineteenth century due to immigrants from China and Japan and later from southeast Asia to Europe and the US. Many temples were established for members to engage in religious ceremonies and rituals. During the 1960s, when young people were searching for new experiences, a significant growth in Buddhism took place. Important Buddhist figures in the West included D. T. Suzuki (1870–1966), who popularized Zen in the West, Thich Nhat Hanh (1926–present), a popular Vietnamese monk, and the Dalai Lama from Tibet. Today there are approximately 1,000 Buddhist meditation centers in the US and Canada and 12.6 percent of the US population believes that Buddhist teachings have influenced their understanding and practice of spirituality (Lewis 2008).

Beliefs and practices

General

It was in the Deer Park in Benares, a city located by the bank of the River Ganges, India, that the Buddha gave his first sermon on the cause and cessation of suffering, now known as "The Four Noble Truths and the Eightfold Path":

> This, monks, is the *Noble Truth of Suffering* (dukkha): birth is suffering; aging is suffering; illness is suffering; death is suffering; presence of objects we hate is suffering; separation from objects we love is suffering; not to obtain what we desire is suffering. In short, the Five Components of Existence are suffering.
>
> This, monks, is the *Noble Truth concerning the Origin of Suffering*: verily, it originates in that craving which causes rebirth, which produced delight and passion, and seeks pleasure now here, now there; that is to say, craving for sensual pleasures, craving for continued life, craving for nonexistence.

This, monks, is the *Noble Truth concerning the Cessation of Suffering*: truly, it is the complete cessation of craving so that no passion remains; the laying aside of, the giving up, the being free from, the harboring no longer of, this craving.

This, monks, is the *Noble Truth concerning the Way which leads to the Cessation of Suffering*: verily, it is this *Noble Eightfold Way*, that is to say, right views, right intent, right speech, right conduct, right means of livelihood, right endeavor, right mindfulness, and right meditation.

(Samyutta Nikaya V:420)

The Buddha teaches that the way out of suffering is through the practice of the Eight Noble Paths. However, common among lay Buddhists is the practice of the Five Precepts that call for abstention from five types of activities: (1) taking life; (2) taking what is not given; (3) sexual immorality; (4) false speech; and (5) intoxication. A more devout Buddhist may seek to practice the Eight Precepts, which include abstention from three additional acts: (1) eating at a wrong time (eat only one meal per day after sunrise and before noon); (2) entertainment and self-adornment such as music, dancing, and jewelry and other types of ornamentation; and (3) luxury and extravagance of all types. It is not uncommon for lay Buddhists to keep the Eight Precepts during the three-month-long Buddhist Lent Day (beginning on the full moon of the eighth lunar month believed to be the day Buddha preached his first sermon).

The teachings of the Buddha may be summarized in three main concepts. These are the belief that life consists of suffering and suffering exists because there is nothing permanent in life, including the self. When one comes to understand that there is no real self, one will find liberation from suffering.

Suffering (dukkha)

"To be is to suffer" is the essential Buddhist assessment of the human existential situation. We are, therefore we suffer. The Buddha taught that birth is painful, decay is painful, disease is painful, death is painful, union with the unpleasant is painful, separation from the pleasant is painful, and unsatisfied cravings are also painful. When we are attached, we set ourselves up for suffering. When we are attached to life, death is painful. When we are attached to others, their departure becomes unbearable. What feeds this attachment is our thirst or our cravings (*tanha*). Buddha teaches that it is the craving desire that leads to becoming. The process of becoming results in the formation of bodily senses (sight, sound, smell, taste, and feeling) leading to gratification. *Tanha* is the fundamental problem of human suffering. It is desire that exacerbates the pain. Most pain we experience in our day-to-day living can be traced back to *tanha*.

But desire may not be bad in itself if not because of the second funda-mental truth in Buddhism, which is impermanence. If our attachment is to that which is permanent, lasting happiness could be conceivable. However, what we desire is always in a state of flux: changing and reconfiguring. If we are attached to something we like and that which we really like remains with us all the time, we may not experience suffering. Unfortunately, this is not the case. To answer this tormenting question pertaining to the cer-tainty of life and of the things we desire, the Buddha points us to the doc-trine of *anicca* or impermanence.

Impermanence (anicca)

"And that which is transient, O monks, is it painful or pleasant?" asked Buddha. "Painful, Master," came the reply. Things we want never remain the same. Life comes and goes. Youth turns to old age. Beauty becomes blemish. Memories deteriorate. Things decay. Nothing is permanent and that is why attachment to such things becomes painful. A river may appear the same, but is it the same river? Contents of the stream, rocks, sand, and pebbles continue to change and reconfigure themselves. Every person goes through the process of continual changes. At every moment we are not the same and yet not the other. We are not the same because our constituent elements change at every moment. Further events that happen in our lives and the information we receive every day are reminders that who we are today are not quite the same as yesterday. At the same time we are not the other because what we are is the result of our past karma (action). Although the appearances of the world and the "I" seem permanent, a careful analysis shows that nature truly is continually changing. All things are operated by the law of causality. A thing is only a state of which the first is said to be the cause of the second because every action has its con-sequence. Existence is only a continuity of changes, each of which is deter-mined by its preexisting conditions. Nothing exists without a condition, and if there is a condition for its existence dissolution is inevitable.

A soul that seeks deliverance must grasp the truth that encompasses the whole of existence – life is *anicca*. And this includes human beings. There is no being but becoming conditioned by certain causes under the opera-tion of the law of causality. Therefore, everything will inevitably end in dissolution. So the Buddha teaches that if our ignorance regarding the world as being permanent leads to attachment and thus suffering, the reverse process, the knowledge of all things being impermanent, can lead to detachment and thus liberation.

No-self (anatta)

The doctrine of *anatta* is the belief that behind the phenomenon we call "self" there is no real self. There is no real "I." What I come to claim as myself is but an illusion caused by the desire to become and to be. The concept of "self" is a perplexing one. What is this "self?" When we move from one social context to another, we could possibly feel and think very differently about ourselves. Further, is it possible that we would perceive ourselves very differently if we were raised in a different place, culture, or socio-economic setting? So who is this being identified by my name?

The Buddha teaches that the illusion that there is a real self is the primary cause for attachment that results in suffering. If there is no real self, there is no need to be attached and when there is no attachment, there is no suffering. This self is nothing but an integration of the four elements (aggregates): earth, water, wind, and fire. Every integration implies the possibility of disintegration. Hence this self is impermanent. It is nothing but a combination of the four basic elements that come together based on the law of karma, the law of cause of effect. In explaining the process of becoming or acquiring the illusion of this self, the Buddha points us to the law of *paticcasamuppada*, or the law of dependent origination, the doctrine that seeks to explain how physical and psychological phenomena are conditionally related with each other. The following are constituent parts of the law of *paticcasamuppada*:

1 Ignorance (*avijja*): Through ignorance arises karma formation. Karma formation can be either unwholesome or wholesome. Unwholesome karma formation refers to one's ignorance that may lead to craving (*tanha*), which results in bad deeds. Wholesome karma formation refers to action based on the right understanding.
2 Karma formation (*sankhara*): Through karma formation arises consciousness.
3 Corporeality and mentality (*nama-rupa*): Through consciousness arise corporeality and mentality, or the physical and the mental aspect of a human being.
4 Six bases (*salayatanam*): Through corporeality and mentality arise six bases. These six bases are: eyes, ears, nose, tongue, body, and mind. These six bases provide contact with the external world.
5 Impression (*phasso*): Through the six bases arise impression. Impression is produced when senses come in contact with the objects of attention.
6 Feeling (*vedana*): Through impression arises feeling. Feeling arises as an immediate concomitance of impression.
7 Craving (*tanha*): Through feeling arises craving. The craving to be detached from that which is unpleasant or be united with that which is pleasant arises from the illusion of the self and the world.
8 Clinging (*upadanam*): Through craving arises clinging.
9 Becoming (*bhavo*): Through clinging arises becoming.
10 Rebirth (*jati*): Through becoming arises rebirth.

11 Old age and death (*jutipaccaya jara-maranam*): Through rebirth arise old age and death, thus suffering.

This doctrine of *paticcasamuppada* helps us realize that in the final analysis there is no self. This self is nothing but a combination of all the aggregates that come together due to karma resulting from ignorance. To understand *anatta* is to know the path leading to the cessation of suffering.

Health and disease

Health is an important aspect in the practice of Buddhism. To understand the Buddhist concept of health requires a perspective on the Buddhist view of life and its meaning in relation to the cause of pain and the way out of the cycle of suffering. Buddhism approaches health from a holistic perspective. Health is the harmonious balance of the body, mind, emotion, and the spiritual dimension, and therefore is not merely the absence of disease. What brings about this harmony is the right understanding of the teachings of Buddha. Hence Buddhist understanding of health is closely connected to spirituality. "According to Buddhism, to be active and healthy, one needs to live a spiritual life" (Hewapathirane 2004: 6). Spirituality is essential because good health derives primarily from correct understanding of the meaning of life and from right practices in accord with the teachings of Buddhism. It requires that one realizes the goal of life, the attainment of enlightenment, through cultivating right understanding, practicing meditation, exerting moderation, and offering compassion. Disease, on the other hand, is the result of ignorance leading to craving desire, impurity, and indulgence that leads to disharmony at the physical, emotional, and spiritual levels. This approach to health points to a strong connection between mind and body. In explaining this relationship, Pinit Ratanakul (2004), professor of religious studies at Mahidol University, affirms that in Buddhism no one can harm us except ourselves. Our thoughts dictate our happiness and through it we can either degrade or improve our wellbeing.

Recent studies on meditation have affirmed the importance of this aspect of Buddhist teaching pertaining to health practice. In 2001, Richard Davidson and Jon Kabat-Zin carried out a study on meditation with a Tibetan Buddhist monk by placing hundreds of sensors on the monk and connecting them to an EEG, a brain-scanning device. When the monk meditated on compassion, the sensors registered a dramatic shift to a state of great joy. Other studies also reveal the positive impact meditation has on the immune system, blood pressure, depression, and stress (Hewapathirane 2004: 7). A study by Somporn Kantharadussadee-Triamchaisri (2004) and associates on the practice of Buddhism among AIDS patients in Thailand shows that Buddhists who practice positive thinking, contentment, compassion, and meditation show significant decreases in their cortisol and stress levels.

This holistic understanding of health does not preclude the utilization of Western medicine. Buddhism promotes every possible means for good health. However, it is important that "disease" is not viewed merely as physical symptoms. As such another fundamental concept contributing to the understanding of health has to be taken into consideration.

While Western medicine treats the body, it lacks the understanding of the way in which one's karma impacts one's health, causing various forms of disease. According to Ratanakul, "Buddhism attributes karma as an important contributing factor to health and disease. In the Buddhist perspective good health is the correlated effect of good karma in the past and vice versa" (Ratanakul 2004: 162). In explaining the role of karma, Ratanakul points to cases of patients who failed to thrive even when the treatment was successful and those who survived even when their medical care was poor. "Karma is created by choices we made in past lives. Health is to be gained by continuing personal efforts in this life. Good deeds lead to good health whereas bad deeds in this and previous lives bring illness" (Ratanakul 2004: 163). While Buddhism recognizes the place of karma in sickness and disease, it is advised that patients do not use this as an excuse for not taking care of their health but to take advantage of every possible means for healing while being mindful of the Buddhist view of life. Because of the emphasis on the mind–body connection, a healthy body plays a significant role in the path toward enlightenment. Through this understanding of the role of karma, it is important that patients learn to accept the reality of disease in their lives and at the same time make positive efforts to comply with medical advice while working on positive karmic formation that will contribute to their overall health and wellbeing in this life and the life to come.

In Buddhism, karma is not viewed strictly on the individual basis. There is also a collective dimension of karma and this may refer to the environmental and social factors that can aggravate or mitigate an individual's health and wellbeing, such as unhealthy or dangerous working conditions. In viewing this collective dimension of karma, it is necessary that governmental agencies play an appropriate role in monitoring and managing healthcare systems and work environments (Ratanakul 2004: 163).

When viewing karma from the context of terminal illness, it becomes even more essential to address the spiritual dimension by promoting cultivation of right understanding, mindfulness, and right practice that will generate positive karma to promote wellbeing, both for the current state and for life to come.

There are a couple of important considerations we need to pay attention to when treating Buddhist patients, such as the issues of diet and the Buddhist's view of abortion. There is generally no restriction when it comes to diet for Buddhists. While vegetarianism is encouraged among all Buddhists, most in the Theravada tradition do not practice vegetarianism. However, a strict Mahayana Buddhist will avoid eating fish and meat. Buddhists who worship *Guan Yin* (the goddess of mercy) do not eat beef. Some Buddhists avoid eating food prepared with onions and garlic due to the belief that they arouse the base senses. Generally Buddhists practice moderation when it comes to food and avoid intoxication of any form since it is one of the Five Precepts.

When the conception of self begins and ends is at times a point of contention in Buddhism. Abortion is an issue in Buddhism because of the reality of this contention. Like other specific issues, abortion is best understood within the broad religious perspective on suffering and the cessation of suffering within the context of life's cycle such as birth, sickness, and death. Life's ultimate goal is the end of suffering and this end takes place when one is no longer caught within the cycle of birth and death under the law of karma. One's birth is determined by one's previous karma (the merits or the lack thereof from one's past life). This fundamental belief forms the basis for the Buddhist approach to ethical issues such as abortion and end-of-life care, including such issues as suicide, euthanasia, and extended life support.

In regard to abortion, the ongoing debates indicate a tendency toward prohibition among Theravada Buddhists and a more accommodating approach among Japanese and Western Buddhists in the US. The very first Buddhist precept is "to abstain from taking life." Hence based on this precept, the practice of abortion is prohibited. Taking the life of the fetus by mothers or physicians, therefore, may result in bad karma. However, the clinical situation is often complex and may require further nuance of this prohibition. In Buddhism, being is nothing but a combination of consciousness and the physical component. When the body lacks consciousness, being does not exist (Barnhart 1997). Therefore, there is no "being" at conception. Being only emerges during a later development. However, there are those who believe that being exists at conception. Regardless, the emergence of the concept of being is not the only consideration in this issue of abortion.

Many Buddhists believe intention must be taken into consideration. Here, it is not purely the act of killing that determines one's karma. If the act is engaged on the basis of compassion, compassion then becomes the source that dictates one's karma. Hence in a situation where abortion may be needed to save the mother's life, this act of abortion may be justifiable when viewed from the perspective of intention and compassion (Hughes 2007: 129). Viewing the issue from the perspective of intention helps to realize that careless and unmindful sexual engagement that may result in pregnancy and hence abortion will certainly result in negative karma.

Another important factor to be considered is the hierarchy of self in Buddhism. Based on the understanding of karma, not all beings have the same moral status. Hence a more fully developed consciousness, such as that of the mother, may hold a higher moral status than that which is less developed, such as the fetus (Hughes and Keown 1995). Losing either the mother or the child is considered tragic, but when practitioners are forced to save one over the other, this Buddhist concept of hierarchy can assist in dealing with difficult decisions. As healthcare providers, it is important to understand Buddhists' approach to abortion and at the very same time be conscious of the various possible interpretations. Understanding patients and making appropriate inquiry can help determine the best course of action. According to the Dalai Lama:

> Of course, abortion, from a Buddhist viewpoint, is an act of killing and is negative, generally speaking. But it depends on the circumstances. If the unborn child will be retarded or if the birth will create serious problems for the parent, these are cases where there can be an exception. I think abortion should be approved or disapproved according to each circumstance.
>
> (Dreifus 1993: 2)

Death and dying

In Buddhism, the dying process is one of the most essential because what happens at this stage plays a significant role in determining life after death. Healthcare professionals can be instrumental in assisting Buddhist patients through this important transition by accommodating their felt needs in the final stage of life. This may be achieved through practicing meditation, reciting Buddhist texts, contemplating the teachings of the Buddha, coming to terms with death, and generating positive thoughts. These practices are possible for patients when the mind is in a state of consciousness. The question is: when does consciousness cease? Some debate exists surrounding the question of when the self ceases to exist because a person, in Buddhist thought, exists only where there is a combination between consciousness and the body (Becker 1990).

There are a number of perspectives on this issue. According to Venerable Mettanando Bhikkhu (1991: 206–7), death occurs in two stages, namely, the lack of high functioning consciousness and the cessation of physical function. When there is an irreversible loss of high-level consciousness (when a patient is in a state of coma or becomes permanently unconscious), it is believed that this consciousness has withdrawn into the interior aspect of the individual. But the death designation is given only when physical death takes place as indicated by the lack of activity of the entire brain, both upper level and lower level:

> Significantly, if the patient is on life-support, such as a respirator, which is doing the job of the lungs although there is no further stimulus to the lungs from the brainstem, the patient can be considered clinically dead. All the reflexes – pupil dilation, swallowing, and breathing

– need to be tested and found negative before the patient can be declared physically dead.

(Mettanando 1991: 206)

Mettanando Bhikkhu makes a distinction between active life termination and withholding treatment. "In a patient for whom the brainstem is no longer driving the bodily functions, life support is no longer needed" because it is in accord with the definition of clinical death (Mettanando 1991: 210). Hence withholding life support is permissible when a person meets the criteria of clinical death.

In Buddhism, there is generally no unifying agreement in relation to euthanasia except that most Buddhists do not practice involuntary euthanasia (termination of life against the will of the patient). There are, however, differing opinions relating to voluntary (when a person makes the decision to end his/her life) and non-voluntary euthanasia (when a person is not capable of making the decision). For most Buddhists, voluntary euthanasia may be perceived as causing bad karma and thus is viewed unfavorably. While there were cases of Buddhist monks voluntarily ending their lives, they took place under exceptional circumstances. Regarding non-voluntary euthanasia, Mettanando believes that termination of life support is possible when all the reflexes such as pupil dilation, swallowing, and breathing are no longer functioning.

When dealing with a deceased patient, Buddhists often let the body rest for two hours before taking any step to transfer the body. Traditionally, a Buddhist monk with incense will lead the body of the deceased to the available transportation and remain in the vehicle until the body arrives at the temple. The length of the funeral service can last up to one week depending on the status and the finances of family members. It is believed that the soul of the deceased will remain near the body for up to three days. The chanting during the service aims at reminding friends and relatives that death is a part of life; it is something we all have to face and accept. The service ends with cremation, a reminder that all our basic elements (earth, water, wind, and fire) will return to their original forms.

Conclusion

Buddhism teaches that our ignorance regarding the true nature of human beings leads to suffering. And the goal of Buddhism is to help people realize the nature of reality and thus be liberated from suffering through acquiring right understanding and through practicing moderation, compassion, meditation, and other beneficial ways of living in accord with the teachings of the Buddha. In matters relating to health, Buddhism emphasizes harmonious balance of the mind, body, emotion, and spirituality and this balance is made possible when one rightly understands the cause of suffering and the ways that can lead to the liberation from the cycle of suffering. Because of

Table 5.1 Dos and don'ts

Dos	Don'ts
1 Pay attention to religious items or sacred threads on patients.	1 Do not remove religious items from patients without permission.
2 Be aware of the role of karma in understanding health and sickness.	2 Do not touch Buddhist monks (for female caregivers) except when they need medical care. Even then, female caregivers should request permission before any form of physical contact.
3 Be aware that clarity of thought prior to death is important since it plays a significant role in determining life after this present death.	
4 Permit the use of religious ceremonies/rituals.	3 Do not offer beef to Mahayana Buddhists who worship Guan Yin (goddess of mercy).
5 Be aware that Buddhist caregivers are reluctant to perform any treatment that they themselves might consider to result in bad karma.	4 Do not invite monks from a tradition different from that of the patient's to perform a religious ceremony.

the importance of the mind–body connection in Buddhism, healthcare providers' awareness of the role of spiritual understanding, spiritual practice, and positive environment in relation to the understanding of karma can help facilitate both physical and spiritual recovery for Buddhist patients.

Case study

Ms. June is a 58-year-old Buddhist woman from Thailand with half a dozen or so of her family now here in the States. Her husband died seven years ago and she had moved here after that critical event. She and her husband had been very close through their years of raising four children (40, 38, 35, and 32 years old) on a small farm in Thailand. She, herself, had been raised by a strong mother after her father died when she was just two years old. Family, farming, and Buddhism were the constants of her life and she depended on each of them to help her manage life well. The differences in context between Thailand and the US for these three constants in her life were dramatic.

Feeling tired for at least a year now, Ms. June tried to help herself feel better by using some over-the-counter pain relievers, sleep aids, and various other things she could afford from her local drug store. She did not want to go to the hospital, in part, because she did not think she could financially afford it, but when her symptoms got worse she went to the emergency room. She was subsequently diagnosed with liver cancer with metastases to other organs. In the hospital for most of the last two months, she was introduced to and received a good deal of help from the palliative care specialists there. Eventually, however, conflict between family and providers began so her family took her home to use their old, tried, and true methods from their family's Buddhist traditions. They held a number of ritual ceremonies in the hope of healing her cancer. Ms. June grew worse and her pain increased so much that her family brought her back to the ER. She had dyspnea and an abdomen pain score of 10/10.

In the hospital Ms. June was intubated and placed on ventilator support. She grew increasingly agitated and restless and at one point even tried to extubate herself. The physician and care team gave Ms. June some morphine to calm her down. This helped stabilize her but the cancer was killing her. The doctor told her family that "She is at the end of her life," and that "She may die at any moment." In a quick and loving response, her children and their monk brought a number of things into the ICU to help her in these last hours. The monk used some cords that he wrapped around her bed, then sprinkled some special sort of water, and he appeared to be praying for her. But as he was doing these special Buddhist ministries, the ICU nurse got very uneasy and finally a unit manager came to Ms. June's room and told the family and the monk to stop what they were doing. Supposedly, these things were disturbing other patients and had some potential to cause infections. This just made Ms. June's family angry. They insisted that the ICU stop treating her and let them take her home.

Questions for reflection

1 Is there anything the ICU could do at this point to help make sure Ms. June has the best care possible while she dies?
2 Is it okay to let a patient like Ms. June go home under these circumstances? It seems unsafe; does the hospital incur any liability for her safety?
3 What is so disruptive about Buddhist prayers/rituals that it would upset an ICU?

Glossary

Anatta   Used to denote a sense of no-self; that is there is no real self. What we term "self" is an illusion.

Annica   Referring to impermanence, this term notes that everything in this life is in the state of impermanence.

Avijja   Refers to our ignorance which ultimately leads us to the cycle of incarnation.

Dukkha   Refers to the sense of suffering that is central to the religion of Buddhism; the Buddha taught that to exist is to suffer.

Paticcasamuppada   The law of dependent origination seeking to explain the cycle of life.

Tanha   Close to the concept of desire. Desire always leads to attachment, and attachment to being.

Bibliography

Barnhart, M. (1997) "Buddhism and the morality of abortion," *Journal of Buddhist Ethics*, vol. 5. Available online at: http://blogs.dickinson.edu/buddhistethics/2010/04/08/buddhism-and-the-morality-of-abortion/ (accessed September 29, 2016).

Becker, C. B. (1990) "Buddhist views of suicide and euthanasia," *Philosophy East and West*, vol. 40: 543–56.

Buddha Dharma Association and BuddhaNet (n.d.). "Statistics on the major branches of Buddhism." Available online at: www.buddhanet.net/e-learning/history/bstats_b.htm (accessed August 10, 2008).

Dreifus, C. (1993) "The Dalai Lama," *New York Times*, November 28, p. 2.

Hewapathirane, D. (2004) "Buddhism, health and wellbeing," *Wisdom*, vol. 9, no. 1: 6–8.

Hughes, J. (2007) "Buddhist bioethics," in Ashcroft, R. E., Dawson, A., Draper, H., and McMillan, J. R. (eds) *Principles of Health Care Ethics*, New York: John Wiley & Sons.

Hughes, J. and Keown, D. (1995) "Buddhism and medical ethics: A bibliographic introduction," *Journal of Buddhist Ethics*, vol. 2. Available online at: www.researchgate.net/publication/239843678_Buddhism_and_Medical_Ethics_A_Bibliographic_Introduction (accessed September 29, 2016).

Kantharadussadee-Triamchaisri, S., Tengtrisron, C. Mahaweerawatana, U., Powatana, A., Permpornsakul, C., and Smitrakasetrin, S. (2004) *Mind-Spiritual Exercise and Healing among HIV/AIDS Patients in Thailand*, Bangkok: Ministry of Health.

Kosmin, B. A. and Keysar, A. (2008) "American Religious Identification Survey," Trinity College, Hartford, CT. Available online at: http://commons.trincoll.edu/aris/files/2011/08/ARIS_Report_2008.pdf (accessed May 31, 2008).

Lewis, G. R. (2008) "Buddhism in America," Buddhist Faith Fellowship of Connecticut, Middletown, CT. Available online at: www.bauddharakshakapadanama.org/sn/pdf/Buddhism%20in%20America.pdf (accessed September 29, 2016).

Liu, J. (2012) "Buddhists," Pew Research Center. Available online at: www.pewforum.org/2012/12/18/global-religious-landscape-buddhist/#ftnrtn12 (accessed May 31, 2016).

Matthews, W. (1999) *World Religions*, 3rd edn, Belmont, CA: Wadsworth.

Mettanando, B. (1991) "Buddhist ethics in the practice of medicine," in Fu, C. W. and Wawrytho, S. A. (eds) *Buddhist Ethics and Modern Society: An International Symposium*, New York: Greenwood.

Ratanakul, P. (2004) "Buddhism, health and disease," *Eubios: Journal of Asian and International Bioethics*, vol. 15: 162–4.

Suggested texts

Coleman, J. W. (2001) *The New Buddhism: The Western Transformation of an Ancient Tradition*, New York: Oxford University Press.

Goleman, D. (2003) *Healing Emotions: Conversations with the Dalai Lama on Mindfulness, Emotions, and Health*, Boston, MA: Shambala.

Halifax, J. (2008) *Being with Dying: Cultivating Compassion and Fearlessness in the Presence of Death*, Boston, MA: Shambala.

Robinson, R. and Johnson, W. (1997) *The Buddhist Religion: A Historical Introduction*, Belmont, CA: Wadsworth.

6 Jainism

Whitny Braun

Introduction

For Jains, time is eternal and cyclical. There is no beginning and there will be no end. The bodies of all life forms are but physical vessels for the eternal soul or the *jīva*. Each soul will move from physical body to physical body again and again throughout time until the soul can limit the amount of *karma* accrued. This allows their soul to break free from the prison of the physical body and float to the top of the universe where it can reside for all time in a formless, blissful, omnipotent state, free from the cycle of reincarnation forever.

In Jainism there is but one maxim that each soul must strive to live by: *Ahiṁsā* or non-violence. Jains strive to pass through this life leaving as little a mark as possible. For Jains, at the end of their lives, they want to leave the world with the slightest "violence footprint" possible.

Demographics

Jains can be found operating in the most elite circles of business, banking, politics, academia, and science. And then you will find them living, by choice, in abject poverty and austerity, seeking to free themselves of all of the trappings of modern life. You rarely find Jains who exist somewhere in the middle.

It is estimated that there are just under five million Jains in the world today, with approximately 4.2 million living in the religion's country of origin, India (Census of India 2011). While the bulk of the Jain population can be found in South Asia, there are sizable diaspora communities across the globe. Africa is home to approximately 20,000 Jains, with major concentrations in Kenya and South Africa (Dundas 2002). Approximately 25,000 Jains reside in the United Kingdom and between 60,000 to 100,000 practicing Jains reside in the United States (Kumar 1996). One of the most prominent diaspora communities (approximately 15,000) is the Jains of Antwerp, Belgium, who are deeply involved in the precious stone trade. Economists estimate that this population now controls up to two-thirds of the wholesale diamond trade in this international commercial hub.

History

The Jain philosophy and religion is believed by its followers to be eternal. There is no creation myth nor is there an apocalyptic future foretold. Instead, Jains believe that civilizations ebb and flow and there have been times in the past and will be times in the future when the truth of Jainism will be known and then disappear into the mists of history again. But the purity and the truth of Jainism will never perish or go extinct. And from time to time throughout the ages twenty-four *Tīrthaṅkaras*, translated as "ford makers" or prophets, appear to share the eternal wisdom of Jain philosophy with humanity. They appear in definite and fixed intervals as perfect beings that serve as great teachers and exemplars (Glasenapp 1999).

In known human history, which Jains understand as just one of an endless series of epochs, twenty-four *Tīrthaṅkaras* have been recorded. The first of these is the mythical figure of Lord Ṛṣabha, also known as Ādinātha (Baya 2007), who may have been a historical figure of the Indus Valley Civilization dating as far back as 3,300 BCE or even predating the civilization, but the earliest of the *Tīrthaṅkaras* that can be reliably dated as a historical figure is the twenty-third, Pārśvanātha, who is believed to have lived circa 877–777 BCE. Whether or not Ādinātha or Pārśvanātha can be credited as being the founders of Jainism in the modern world is debatable. From the Jain perspective, there can be no founder of Jainism as it is an eternal truth and not the teachings of one man. From the perspective of the historical academy, the title of founder of the faith traditionally belongs to a man who lived from 599–527 BCE known as Mahāvīra.

There is little doubt that Mahāvīra was a historical figure. Not only is his existence documented in many Jain writings but he is also referenced in Buddhist scriptures as a contemporary of Gautama Buddha (Glasenapp 1999). He was born Vardhamāna, the son of a *Kṣatriya* named Siddhārtha and his wife Triśalā in the Kuṇḍagrāma, located in the present-day Indian state of Bihar. His father, as *Rājā*, provided him with a life of privilege and opulence, a marriage to a princess who bore him a daughter, and all of the luxuries he desired.

By his thirtieth year of life he renounced his royal privilege and set off on his own (Jaini 1998). He first traveled to an area of wilderness called Śandavana and fasted for two and a half days under an Aśoka tree. According to the Śvetambara tradition, he donned robes of *deva-dūṣya* or divine cloth and proceeded to pull out his hair in five tufts in the ritual known as *kesá-loca* (Jaini 1998). He then shed his robes so as to purge himself of any possessions and became a nude itinerant monk wandering the countryside.

He first joined the order of ascetics believed by historians to have been founded on the teachings of Pārśvanātha near his hometown but found that they did not live in austere enough conditions and so chose to wander on his own. For twelve years he walked the area of the Ganges River Basin and was the subject of scorn, ridicule, and mockery for his nudity and ascetic practices. But, by the end of his twelfth year of itinerant preaching, he attained omniscience (*kevala jñana*) while sitting under a tree on the banks of the Ṛjupālikā River. It was in this moment of conquering his passions and mental frailties that he earned the title of Mahāvīra, or "the great hero," as he assumed the role of an *arihant*, a venerable person who would become the twenty-fourth *Tīrthaṅkaras*.

Upon accession to the role of *Tīrthaṅkaras*, he made it his duty to revive the teachings of Pārśvanātha. He set out on foot through the countryside of Bihar and for the next thirty years preached to both men and women of all walks of life. It is believed that he died in 527 BCE at the age of seventy-two after having taken the vow of *Sallekhanā* and achieved *mokṣa* (complete liberation), and ascended to the apex of the universe to exist for all eternity in the abode of the *Siddhas* (*Siddhaloka*) in a perfect, formless, genderless state.

According to tradition, Mahāvīra had converted 14,000 monks, 36,000 nuns, 159,000 laymen and 318,000 lay women to the Jain system of belief by the time of his death (Glasenapp 1999). It is commonly believed that Mahāvīra passed away within the lifetime of the Buddha and in the years following both of their deaths, Jainism and Buddhism emerged as the premiere Śramanic faiths of the Vedic period in northern India.

The Jain community split into two main sectarian groups: *Digambaras* and *Śvetāmbaras*. The *Digambaras* are the "sky clad" sect known for their male ascetics who give up clothing and live as itinerant monks in the nude. The *Digambaras* are further divided into at least three distinct sectarian groups: the *Digambara Terapatha* of Śuddhāmnāya, the *Bispanth*, and the *Samaiyā* (Jain 1999). The *Śvetāmbaras* are the "white clad" sect known for their ascetics wearing simple white robes and often a cloth across their mouths called a *muphatti* to prevent the accidental inhalation of microscopic life. The *Śvetāmbaras* are further divided into sub-sects: the *Murtipujaka Deravasi*, the *Sthānakavāsi*, and the *Terapanthi*. There are several differences in the beliefs and practices of these two sects but perhaps the most notable, besides the differences in their appearance and attitudes toward idol worship and the historical timeline, is that *Digambaras* hold that all twenty-four of the *Tīrthaṅkaras* were men. Additionally, they believe that only men can achieve *mokṣa*, whereas the *Śvetāmbaras* believe that women can achieve *mokṣa*, entering the *siddha* state directly from the form of a human woman. The *Śvetāmbaras* believe that the nineteenth *Tīrthaṅkara* was a woman named Māllīnātha (Jaini 1998). It is possible that because of this *Śvetāmbaras*' belief that women can achieve *mokṣa*, more *Śvetāmbara* women are recorded as engaging in *Sallekhanā*.

There is debate as to how the schism between the two main sects in Jainism came about. One theory is that the once homogenous population split about two centuries after the death of Mahāvīra around the year 290 BCE when the ācārya Śri Bhadrabāhu migrated along with 12,000 ascetics and lay followers from Pāṭaliputra to the state of Karnataka in the South of India in a desperate attempt to avoid a famine. It is said that Bhadrabāhu passed away before a return to Bihar was possible and when a few followers did return they found that many of the practices of their original community had changed under the leadership of Sthūlabhadra, including the wearing of clothing. Unable to accept these changes, the group that had left Pāṭaliputra under Bhadrabāhu became the *Digambaras* and those who followed the leadership of Sthūlabhadra became the *Śvetāmbaras* (Jaini 1998). This division was cemented at the Council of Vallabhi in the fifth century CE (Kelting 2003).

Beliefs and practices

General

One aspect of Jain doctrine that distinguishes it from most other religions is that in the last three millennia it has experienced very little dogmatic development when compared to the Abrahamic or even other Dharmic traditions (Glasenapp 1999). After Mahāvīra's death, his disciples, the *Gaṇadharas*, recorded his teachings and a lineage of Jain scholars was established that produced the works that continue to form the corpus of the Jain canons. Thus, the practices prescribed for the aspirant who wishes to achieve a good death have remained almost unchanged through the centuries.

Jain soteriology can only be understood in the context of Jain cosmology. Jainism does not espouse that the universe (*loka*) was created by an intelligent, divine being but rather describes the universe as an eternal, physical constant, made up of six *dravya* or substances that also have always been and always will be. These *dravya* are: sentient beings or souls (*jīva*), non-sentient matter (*pudgala*), energy of motion (*dharma*), the principle of rest (*adharma*), space (*ākāśa*), and time (*kāla*).

The cosmos is a giant space where the abode of the liberated souls, the heavens where the gods reside, the middle world, which contains the realm of men, and the seven levels of hell exist. This universe is conceptualized in the shape of a man with arms bent, resting on the hips and feet planted apart. Outside of this *loka*, there is nothing but a giant void filled with strong winds (Dundas 2002).

Again, this *loka* is not the work of a conscious, divine entity. It has no beginning and no end and is an eternal physical cosmos, thus there is no eschatological view in Jainism. In the *loka*, there are three realms that exist below the supreme abode of the *Siddhas*: the infernal, terrestrial, and celestial.

Only those *jīva* who are born into the realm of men can theoretically hope to strive for deliverance from their earthly physical form.

The infernal realm or *Naraka* exists at the bottom of the *loka*, where there are seven levels of hell. As one goes deeper through the levels of hell, the geographical expanse of each gets broader, and the beings that exist in these realms are characterized by a dark soul coloring (*parināma*) and commit violence against each other, causing pain and suffering. Below the bottommost hell there are no forms of life (Shah 2000). The beings that exist in these hells are not born in the same way that humans are born in the middle earth. They are oddly born by spontaneously manifesting from holes in the walls and falling into the hell. These beings are hermaphrodites and fully conscious of their suffering (Shah 2000).

Located above the hellish realms is the circular middle realm known as middle *loka* or *Madhyaloka* and in the center of this terrestrial realm there are numerous oceans and countless continents rising from the waters. The continents derive their names as a result of their unique characteristics. The oceans are named for the liquids that their water resembles (Shah 2000). Rising from the center of this middle earth is Mount Meru. The middle world has a central continent of *Jambūdvīpa*, translated as "The Island of the Roseapple Tree," forming with the adjacent continent of *Dhātakīkhaṇḍa* and half of the continent nearest to it, *Puskaradvīpa*, to create the abode of humankind (Dundas 2002). *Jambūdvīpa* is surrounded by an imposing wall built entirely of diamonds and a large lotus-terrace with ponds built from precious stones. There is also said to be a large gate wrought from gold and jewels with four entry points protected by deities (Glasenapp 1999). Outside these gates is the abode of humankind.

Those who conquer *saṁsāra* and travel to the abode of the *Siddhas* do so from the abode of humankind. However, there is another realm above the middle realm where the celestial beings reside.

Above the middle world is a series of heavens, which increase in size and brightness and beauty, and where gods and goddesses exist. This realm is called the *devloka*. These gods are divided into four *nikāyas* or species: *Bhavanapati*, *Vyantara*, *Jyotiṣka*, and *Vaimānika* (Glasenapp 1999). While the hellish beings are greyish in color, the heavenly beings enjoy light bodily colors. Among the *Vaimānkas* the gods have a yellow bodily color and those gods who live in the third up to the fifth heavens have a red form, while all gods residing in the sixth heaven up to the *sarvārthasiddha* have white bodies (Glasenapp 1999).

Ultimately gods and goddesses must be reborn in the middle world as men or women to continue on the path to *mokṣa* so their time in the celestial realm is somewhat bittersweet in that they will need to leave that heavenly abode to continue on their spiritual journey. Some of these gods and goddesses can experience sexual enjoyment but that enjoyment will ultimately lead to their fall. The greater the intensity of the sexual passion, the greater their mental desire and the greater the desire, the harder it is to satisfy it. Thus a struggle ensues for the god that will ultimately result in the god being reborn in human form. The higher up in the levels of heaven a god resides, the larger their physical form, the longer their life, and the more pleasure they feel while the less arrogance they possess (Shah 2000).

Above the heavens and at the end of the upward climb up the levels of the *loka* is the *Īsatprāgbhāra*, or "slightly curving place" (Dundas 2002: 91) where the liberated souls exist, experiencing pure knowledge, energy, and bliss, having broken through the cycles of *saṁsāra*, freeing themselves from the pain of birth, death, and rebirth.

Health and disease

In Jain philosophy, as long as the soul remains in its mundane unenlightened existence decay, disease, and death are certain. Life is not thought of as a pleasant experience. The *Uttarādhyayanasūtra* says that "birth, death, decay and disease are sorrows, the mundane existence itself is full of sorrow, where the living beings feel miserable." Further, the *Ādi Śaṅkarācārya* says that repeated births and deaths, the process known as *saṁsāra*, and lying in the wombs of mothers is very painful.

The death of humans and animals occurs when the being has reached the quantum of life allotted to it by its *karma*. This death occurs as a result of a specific cause known as an *upakrama* but for gods and hellish beings death takes place spontaneously and the *jīva* is carried along on its spiritual journey by the force of *anupūrvināmakarma* to the next place of its rebirth. This time between death and rebirth is infinitesimally short and known as *vigrahakāla* (Glasenapp 1999).

The ultimate spiritual desire for the Jains has been to find a way to be set free from the physical pain and fear that is inherent in the form of a living being. Life is characterized by fear and suffering with the end result of death and to be free of this cycle of violence and pain is the supreme wish. The Jain *Tīrthaṅkaras* developed and shared a unique way to overcome this fear and the accompanying misery of life by teaching a practice which allowed a person to approach death voluntarily in a state of equanimity. They prescribed a ritual in which a person sheds the *karma* that weighs down their soul and achieves *moksha* or liberation of the soul. This concept is unique to the Jain philosophy and is referred to as *Samādhimaraṇa*, the peaceful death, and the ritual itself is popularly known as *Sallekhanā* (Glasenapp 1999).

Ultimately each soul needs to purge itself of *karma* in order to achieve spiritual deliverance or *mokṣa*. But there are steps on the journey to *mokṣa*. The individual should strive for right belief, right knowledge, and right conduct. By striving to perfect the soul, the individual can work toward achieving enlightenment and becoming a *kevalin*. However, being a *kevalin* and enjoying omniscience does not immediately seal one's fate as having achieved liberation. Upon attaining enlightenment, the individual may live for quite some time engaging in mental and physical activities such as walking, preaching, and meditation. However, no new *karma* is accrued at this time and the individual is not committing any acts of violence (Dundas 2002).

Paul Dundas explains the next step in the process of moving from enlightenment to liberation as follows:

> It is necessary for life karma to run its course before final deliverance can be gained. From the time of the scriptural texts, Jain theoreticians claimed that is might be necessary for the enlightened person, or *kevalin*, to perform an expulsion (*samudghāta*) of karmic particles in order to equalize experience karma, which has been generally bound more intensely than any other type, with life karma. This strange process is effected by the kevalin expanding the *jīva* for the short duration of eight instants, to the height and width of the *loka* in a variety of temporarily assumed shapes, whereupon, after ejecting karmic particles in the same way as dust is shaken off an open sheet which is then refolded, it subsequently returns to the confines of the human body. This ensures that the non-harming karmas will quickly reach their end and the *kevalin* then starts to run down the operation of the mind, body and speech until all natural functioning ceases.
>
> (2002: 104)

The *kevalin* then articulates five verses, and the four non-harming *karmas* disappear. The *jīva* becomes free from its body or physical prison and then ascends through the *loka* instantaneously and enters the abode of the *Siddhas* at the top of the universe. Here in the abode of the *siddhas* the *jīva* will exist in a perfect, peaceful, genderless state experiencing only bliss.

Sallekhanā, Santhārā, or *Samādhimaraṇa,* all terms used in the Jain religion to describe a ritualistic voluntary and peaceful death, are discussed in the Jain canonical texts. This end-of-life ritual is regarded as one of the most prestigious rites of passage in the Jain code of conduct. Jain canonical lore is full of prescriptions for and instances of individuals, both monastics and laity, choosing this journey to voluntary death in order to culminate their spiritual journey in this lifetime. It serves as the supreme expression of Jain faith and as a means to reach liberation of the soul.

Death and dying

In the broadest sense of Jain philosophy, an eternal soul (*jīva*) is subject to the cycle of birth, death, and rebirth (*saṁsāra*). When in a physical form, particularly a human form, the worth of the body that houses the soul is based on utility. The physical body is a tool or the conduit by which the soul seeks out knowledge and enlightenment and proceeds on its spiritual journey. When the physical body begins to fail and is more of a burden than an asset the Jain canons teach that the enlightened aspirant is best served by accepting that their body is but a temporary vessel and that death is a natural progression and thus it is preferable to embrace death rather than hang on to life. The Jain canons in essence suggest that rather than allowing the grim specter of death to stalk you, you as the aspirant give up life-sustaining practices such as eating and drinking and meet death with a posture of openness. And in this psychological acceptance of death you adopt a position or attitude of equanimity toward death.

The *Tattvārtha Sutra*, compiled in the fifth century BCE represents the earliest known compendium of Jain doctrinal beliefs. The author of this massive work was the chief disciple of Lord Mahāvīra, a man named *Umāsvati*, who created a "handbook for understanding the meaning of the basic truths" (Glasenapp 1999: 126), in which he describes fourteen stages through which a soul must travel to reach the end point of *mokṣa* or liberation upon death. These fourteen phases are known as the *Guasthāna* or "levels of virtue" and are likened to the rungs of a ladder (Jaini 1998). One may climb up or down on the ladder depending on one's actions but in order to achieve the ultimate goal of transcending the cycle of *saṁsāra*, a *jīva* must at some point move sequentially up the ladder, through the fourteen stages.

Each higher stage moves the practitioner from various states of ignorance, passion, bad conduct, and more *karma* to states of omniscience, less passion, perfect conduct, and decreasing amounts of *karma* until there is no *karma* left at all. This path to perfection is sometimes called the "path of purification" (Jaini 1998: 141).

Until omniscience is gained at the top of the ladder upon becoming a *kevalin*, a person cannot claim to know the whole truth of reality, so that every assertion must be qualified as a partial truth. True understanding of the nature of existence remains elusive to all until omniscience is achieved.

The linguistic origin of the word *Sallekhanā* in Prakrit has the commonly accepted definition of "properly thinning out the passions of the body" (Jaini 1998). It is the combination of the prefix *sam* meaning "proper" and *lekhanā*, which translates as "reducing the physical body." Any Jain who is faced with ailments can approach their guru and express their wish to take the vow of *Sallekhanā*. They do so by saying the words:

> Please instruct me sir. I have come forward to seek ... *Sallekhanā*, (the vow of) which will remain in force as long as I live. I am free of all doubts and anxieties in this matter. I renounce, from now until the moment of my last breath, food and drink of all kinds.
>
> (Jaini 1998: 229)

Assuming that permission is granted, the person either decides independently or consults with their physician as to the approximate amount of time he or she has left to live and then develops a program of fasting to coincide with their vow of *Sallekhanā*. While the philosophical rationale surrounding *Sallekhanā* has remained virtually unchanged through the centuries, one adaption that is evolving is that more Jains are consulting their physician for an opinion and assistance in formulating a timetable for *Sallekhanā*. At any time and at any stage along the human wellness spectrum, an individual may begin the ritual. Ideally, the *Sallekhanā* undertaken by the perfectly healthy person of sound mind and body is the most spiritually rewarding form, and is known as *Prāyopagamana* (Madhukar 1982).

A member of the laity who accepts the vow gives up all personal relationships and possessions. He or she forgives all and asks for the pardon of all their sins (Sogani 2005: 231). During this period all negative emotion should be eliminated. It must also be understood that if they are committing to *Sallekhanā* in response to a terminal diagnosis that should their disease be cured, or their diagnosis found to be incorrect, the vow of *Sallekhanā* may not be rescinded.

Sallekhanā is typically done in the family home or in a fasting hall known as a *dharmaśala*. Historically though, such as in the case of Lord Mahāvīra, it was undertaken in a remote space in nature. While a person practices *Sallekhanā* they have no worldly responsibilities. They turn all property over to their family and sequester themselves to avoid distraction. Relatives often publicize the event by taking out ads in local newspapers. When the person eventually dies, it is not uncommon for the body to be ornately decorated and paraded through the community before cremation.

The practice of ritual suicide by starvation is not unique to the Jains (Keown 2001). What is distinctive is that it is so entrenched in the culture and is practiced on such a consistent basis (Laidlaw 2005). Not every Jain takes the vow of *Sallekhanā*, but all Jains have the option available to them. What makes *Sallekhanā* more remarkable is that while this death ritual is prescribed as a necessary step on the path to liberation all Jains know that if they take the vow, it will not result in liberation for them at this time. At best they hope that making the choice to take the vow of *Sallekhanā* results in reincarnation in a better form and place in the next life.

Samādhimaraṇa, Sallekhanā, and Santhārā

While the terms *Samādhimaraṇa* and *Sallekhanā* are frequently used interchangeably they have distinctly different grammatical and conceptual nuances. *Samādhimaraṇa* is a state of being, a peaceful death, and a dispassionate end. It is the experience of death itself, a singular point in time. *Sallekhanā* is a vow followed by a process; a ritual journey one embarks on to achieve *Samādhimaraṇa* (Baya 2007).

The peaceful death and the journey toward achieving it were perhaps developed as a response to the truth written in the *Daśavaikālika Sutra*, which says ever so simply, "Everyone wants to live and none wants to die" (*Daśavaikālika*, 6.10). This may be true enough but as death is inevitable the great Jain thinkers had to philosophize a response to this existential woe. Thus, they sought to create and apply a moral value and ethical framework to the process of death and dying and developed a code that prescribes conquering the fear of death in a fully engaged manner.

This process of accepting death, of psychologically preparing oneself to voluntarily end one's life, should ideally result in the person looking back on a life of piety and therefore having no fear because they are assured of a good reincarnation. The *Tattvārthasūtra* tells that the aspirant should think, "I have followed the path of virtue and thus I do not fear death" (*Tattvārthasūtra*, 7.22). Conversely one who has lived a sinful life full of worldly attachments dies fretfully, fearing death for fear of being reborn in hellish circumstances or as an animal (*Āturpratyākhyān*, 63).

The Jain emphasis on the primary importance of conduct in achieving spiritual liberation has led to the development of a highly rigorous code of monastic practices and a very stringent code of conduct for its laity. Severe penance as a means of purging accumulated *karma* from the soul is prescribed for all followers of the Jain philosophy. The volumes of the *Ardhamāgadhī* canonical works are filled with the concept and detailed procedural descriptions for the attainment of *Samādhimaraṇa* by *Sallekhanā*.

There are linguistic nuances to the terms *Sallekhanā* and *Santhārā* and there are distinctions in how they should be used and the spiritual implications they connote.

Sallekhanā

In the *Sthānāṅga Vṛtti*, the *Ācārya* Abhayadevasūri said that *Sallekhanā* is, "The activity by which the body is weakened and passions are overcome" (*Maranassabihemi*, 63). The *Jñātā-dharmakathā-sūtra* *Vṛtti* echoes the same definition (*Jñātādharmakathāṅga* 1/1 *Vṛtti*). Other works give a slightly different linguistic allusion, describing *Sallekhanā* as the "peeling off of the passions" of the body and the forfeiting bodily strength in order to strengthen the spirit. To weaken the physical body is *Dravya Sallekhanā* while to overcome the passions of the body is *Bhāva Sallekhanā*. Since Jain thought considers the body a prison for the soul and the passions like the chains that hold the soul in its prison, it is of paramount importance in Jain belief to weaken these two entities in order to liberate the soul.

Sallekhanā is a continuing practice aimed at weakening the body externally and the passions internally. Thus, *Sallekhanā* can actually be an open-ended form of preparatory penance that trains the aspirant to embrace the final act of death but does not necessarily have to end in death. The penance in and of itself is a spiritually rewarding ritual. The positive death that results from *Sallekhanā* is then called *Santhārā* or *Samādhimaraṇa*. This sets it apart linguistically and conceptually from *Santhārā*, which is just death. Also, the option of specific periods of time in which to take *Sallekhanā*, such as twelve years, twelve months, or twelve weeks, proves that it is an open-ended penance that is not always meant to end in death.

The *Ācārāṅga* is categorical in stating that a monk must gradually reduce his food intake and weaken his body in order to prepare for the end-practice of *Santhārā* when and only when he feels that his body has become incapacitated due to various reasons and he is unable to bear it any longer. According to the *Ācārya Samantabhadra*, *Antima Māraṇāntika Sallekhanā* must be practiced in cases of acute affliction like famine, extreme old age, and incurable disease (Baya 2007).

Santhārā

Santhārā, unlike the open-ended ritual that *Sallekhanā* can be, is the end practice of embracing voluntary death and end the life. The three types of rigor (*Bhaktapratyākhyāna*, *Inginī*, and *Padapoapagamana*) associated with the final moments of life are associated with the category of *Santhārā*.

Santhārā is considered to be the aspirations of the devout Jain come to fruition after lifelong penance (*Mṛtyu Mahotsava*, 2). But it should be noted that this rigorous lifelong penance is only useful if the aspirant has attained equanimity of mind at the time of death (*Mṛtyu Mahotsava*, 23).

Sallekhanā may be a relatively obscure practice, used by very small subsets of the population, but because of its dramatically different approach to the ending of a person's life it is a potentially problematic ritual for the allopathic medical community to rationalize. Allopathic medicine has evolved to place sustaining life as the major ethical and moral objective of its practitioners.

While *Sallekhanā* is a ritual native to India, its practice is spreading to the United States (Shah 2013). Though official numbers are unknown, conversations with members of the Jain community reveal that it is increasing in frequency as more Jains immigrate to the United States. In order for the United States to maintain cultural pluralism, the medical community needs to become familiar with the rules, rationale, and rituals associated with this practice in order to offer Jain patients in the clinical setting effective holistic care and possibly prevent the abuse of the practice of *Sallekhanā*.

The perception of *Sallekhanā* to an outsider may be macabre. The idea of a person abstaining from food and water may seem torturous and abusive. It would be natural for someone such as a physician, unfamiliar with the practice, to immediately come to the conclusion that the person enduring the fast is experiencing discomfort. Then, based on the default position that a healthcare provider offers comfort to a person who is ailing, the physician may try to offer comfort in the form of nutrition or hydration. And when the person declines that offer the physician may interpret the person's choice to fast to death as being symptomatic of mental incapacity. In which case a conflict may arise between the physician, the patient, and the state as to whether that person is practicing religious freedom or demonstrating decisional incapacity that requires they be protected from themselves.

Non-Jain clinicians both in India and in the United States can lay the groundwork for an inter-faith and inter-cultural dialogue that could facilitate a reconciliation of the American healthcare system's largely Christian-inspired bioethics with the Jain concept of right knowledge and practice. Would it not break the principle of "do no harm" to deprive a person who believes that their soul will be wounded and their future lives negatively impacted by being prevented from engaging in their religiously sanctioned, ideal form of death?

Conclusion

The normative ethics of *Sallekhanā* constitute a larger and more complicated issue. For healthcare professionals, *Sallekhanā* is an ethically and morally troubling practice. If *Sallekhanā* is ever used as a means of coercing the elderly, infirm, or simply unwanted members of the society into suicide, the practice is unquestionably wrong. However, if *Sallekhanā* is a religious ritual and an exercise in personal and patient autonomy that brings comfort to the dying in their final days, then *Sallekhanā* may also be an ethically defensible path toward death.

To outlaw *Sallekhanā* would be unethical as a violation of the right to religious freedom guaranteed not only in the constitutions of the United States and India but by Article 18 of the Universal Declaration of Human Rights. However, in the interest of protecting vulnerable members of the community, both the Jain and global communities' attention must be drawn to *Sallekhanā* to prevent its abuse. For the sake of delivering culturally appropriate counsel and treatment to those members of the Jain community seeking healthcare, it is imperative that medical professionals familiarize themselves with the rules, rituals, and rationale of *Sallekhanā*.

Ultimately the argument must be put forth that within Jain communities – whether in India or in the United States or in any liberal democracy – the moral presumption should be that *Sallekhanā* is a valid religious ritual of dying and therefore should be legally protected. However, the legal sanctioning of *Sallekhanā* should only occur when chosen by a rational person. Given that *Sallekhanā* is sometimes abused, the person contemplating *Sallekhanā* should be advised of the availability of medical treatment for the condition precipitating consideration of *Sallekhanā*, if such treatment exists, and of the right to forgo *Sallekhanā* if the person is experiencing pressure or coercion in any form.

Table 6.1 Dos and don'ts

Dos	Don'ts
1 Do encourage a Jain to be open about their faith.	1 Do not encourage a Jain to eat meat or take antibiotics.
2 Do encourage Jains to ask for a quiet space to practice meditation.	2 Do not encourage a Jain to take heroic measures to extend their lifespan.
3 Do encourage a Jain to ask for assistance from a palliative care specialist.	3 Do not attempt to encourage a Jain to eat if they are fasting.
4 Do acknowledge that Jains do not view *Sallekhanā* as suicide.	4 Do not encourage a Jain to practice abortion or engage in any other act that could be construed as violence.
5 Do acknowledge that some Jains may choose to pursue more aggressive treatment and forgo Sallekhanā.	5 Do not assume that all Jains will choose Sallekhanā.

Case study

A thirty-six-year-old married mother of two was diagnosed with stage 3 ovarian cancer. Her physicians explained to her that her best chance for survival would likely lie in having a hysterectomy followed by radiation and chemotherapy.

After discussing her prognosis and treatment options with her family, the young mother told her physicians that she would like to forgo treatment and instead move forward with taking the vow of *Sallekhanā* and slowly fasting to death.

Initially her primary care physician felt that her reaction to the diagnosis was the result of depression and a general sense of hopelessness and despair following the news of her diagnosis. At the next appointment, the physician wanted to speak to the woman and her husband about how to move forward with treatment.

The woman's husband, who was also a Jain, wanted his wife to pursue whatever treatment options were available. The woman explained that as a Jain she felt her body was just a physical vessel for her soul and now that her physical body was failing her she did not want to begin down a path of committing acts of *hiṃsā* or violence in the form of taking heroic measures to prolong her life.

The hysterectomy would require that she take antibiotics following the surgery. Because Jains believe that all life forms have eternal souls that are of equal value, she believed that taking antibiotics was in essence a form of genocide as she would be killing the millions of bacteria that live in her body. Furthermore, the chemotherapy and radiation would kill other microbial life forms in her body aside from the cancer cells. Assuming the hysterectomy and subsequent chemotherapy and radiation proved successful, she discussed how she knew she would need to take hormone replacements and many of the hormone replacements on the market are derived from porcine (pig) and equine (horse) cellular sources. As a vegan and deeply believing Jain, she would not take medicines that contained animal by-products.

Despite her husband's desire for his wife to undergo the treatment schedule, her physicians prescribed the woman was resolute that she would take the vow of *Sallekhanā*. In the following months, she began to experience such debilitating pain from the cancer that her husband worked with her physicians to arrange hospice care in their home. In the last month of her life, she asked her husband to move framed photos of her children a few feet further away from the side of her bed each day until they were completely out of sight. She then asked her husband to stop visiting her in her room and allow her to pass away without feeling any emotional attachment. When the pain became debilitating her husband intervened and, despite the admonitions against using any kind of medicines during the fasting ritual, had her placed on a morphine drip so that she could pass away more comfortably.

Nine months after receiving her diagnosis, the woman passed away in her home, not from the cancer but from renal failure induced by her refusal to eat or drink. She was cremated, as is the custom in Jain culture.

Questions for reflection

1 Is it the place of a physician to question a patient of faith's motives in choosing to forgo treatment for terminal cancer?
2 Does a young mother have an obligation to honor the wishes of her husband and pursue treatment for the sake of the well-being of her children in spite of her spiritual beliefs?

Glossary

Ācārya A spiritual preceptor; the head of a monastic order.

Ahiṁsā Non-violence; the chief of the five vows of the *vratas*.

Digambara Jain sect; translates as "sky-clad"; *Digambara* Jain male ascetics are nude.

Hiṁsā Violence.

Jīva Soul; one of the five basic substances that make up the matter of the universe.

Karma 1. Action. 2. Karma-matter or particles of Karma *Pudgala Vargaṇā*. 3. Karmic encumbrance earned through one's mental, vocal, or physical activities.

Kevalin One who is omniscient.

Mokṣa   Emancipation; liberation.

Sallekhanā   External and internal penance to weaken the body and passions before undertaking the practice of *Samādhimaraṇa*.

Samādhi   The state of equanimity of mind or that of being peaceful, calm, and tranquil; psychic disposition of spiritual peace.

Saṁsāra   The world of transmigration; the process of birth, death, and rebirth.

Santhārā   1. Literally, the grass bed on which the *kṣapaka* lies for his end practice. 2. Metaphorically, the practice of *Samādhimaraṇa*.

Siddha   An emancipated soul.

Śramanic   The religious traditions which do not believe in a supreme deity, such as Jainism and Buddhism, unlike Hinduism, which believes in a supreme divinity over the universe and is thus Bhramanic.

Śvetāmbara   Jain sect; translates as "white clad."

Tīrthaṅkaras   The supreme religious leaders of Jainism; "Fordmaker."

Bibliography

Baya, D. S. (2006) "Relevance of Sallekhana in Today's Society and Euthanasia," *Conference paper delivered at the International Summer School for Jain Studies*, Jaipur, India.

Baya, D. S. (2007) *Death with Equanimity: The Pursuit of Immortality*, Jaipur: Prakrit Bharati Academy.

Census of India (2011) *Census of India: Religion*, New Delhi, India: Registrar General and Census Commissioner of India.

Dundas, P. (2002) *The Jains*, The Library of Religious Beliefs and Practices, London: Routledge.

Glasenapp, H. von (1999) *Jainism: An Indian Religion of Salvation*, New Delhi, India: Motilal Banarsidass Publishers.

Jain, J. P. (1999) *Religion and Culture of the Jains*, New Delhi: Bharatiya Jnanpith.

Jaini, P. S. (1998) *The Jaina Path of Purification*, New Delhi, India: Motilal Banarsidass Publishers.

Kelting, M. W. (2003) "Good wives, family protectors: Writing Jain laywomen's memorials," *Journal of the American Academy of Religion*, vol. 71, no. 3: 637–657.

Keown, D. (2001) *Buddhism and Bioethics*, London: Palgrave.

Kumar, B. (1996) *Jainism in America*, New Delhi: Jain Humanities Press.

Laidlaw, J. (2005) "A life worth leaving: Fasting to death as telos of a Jain religious life," *Economy & Society*, vol. 34, no. 2: 178–199.

Madhukar, M. (1982) *ĀcārāṇGa*, Beawar, India: Āgamas Prakasana Samiti.

Shah, A. K. (2013) "Global peace ambassador Mr. Keshavji Rupshi Shah, passes on – 21 June," *Diverse Ethics*. Available online at: www.diverseethics.com/newsletters/?y=2013&id=104 (accessed January 10, 2016).

Shah, J. B. (ed.) (2000) *Pt Sukhlalji's Commentary on Tattvartha Sutra of Vacaka Umasvati*, 2nd edn, Ahmedabad, India: L. D. Institute of Indology.

Sogani, K. C. (2005) *Jainism: Ethico – Special Perspective*, Rajasthan: Jaina Vidya Samsthana.

7   Chinese religions

Kwang-Hee Park

To be able under all circumstances to practice five things constitutes perfect
virtue; these five things are gravity, generosity of soul, sincerity, earnestness
and kindness.

Confucius

Manifest plainness, embrace simplicity, reduce selfishness, have a few desires.

Lao-Tzu

Introduction

Chinese religion is a diverse and complex system of traditions that were
developed throughout 2,000 years. Confucianism, Taoism, Buddhism, and
popular folk religions are the four main traditions that have formulated
the core of Chinese thought, cosmology, religious beliefs, and practice.
Confucianism served as an ordering ethical principle to shape Chinese
social roles and responsibilities. As a mystical religio-philosophical tradition, Taoism pursued longevity in interaction with nature. Buddhism,
though a foreign import, expanded and deepened traditional religious
beliefs and spiritual practices. The popular folk religions embraced diverse
aspects of Taoism, Buddhism, and Confucianism and provided a practical
guideline to promote prosperity and happiness in this world. Chinese religion is composed of practical and mysterious traditions that laid the
foundation to create relational harmony between heaven and earth,
between human beings and nature, and between the past and the present.

This chapter explores the beliefs and practices of traditional Chinese
religion, primarily focusing on Confucianism and Taoism as indigenous
traditions that influenced the formation of unique Chinese health beliefs
and practices. In addition to these matters, the chapter introduces Chinese
medicine as the integration of Chinese health beliefs and health practices
and its clinical cautions. The practice of Chinese medicine in China and
Taiwan is different from that of Traditional Chinese Medicine (TCM) in
the United States. There is a limitation in the scope of practice of TCM in
the United States compared to China or Taiwan.

Demographics

Traditional Chinese religions – Confucianism, Taoism, universism (a natural philosophy), divination practice, and Buddhist elements – are widely practiced in 60 countries around the world with more than 225 million adherents. According to Pew Global Attitudes Project conducted in 2006, 31 percent of the population in China considers religion to be important in their lives. It is interesting to note that the 2005 survey finds that approximately three of five Chinese believe in some form of supernatural phenomena associated with Confucianism and folk religion, such as fortune and fate, Jade Emperor, immortal souls, and ghosts. This suggests that popular religion may have permeated Chinese religious beliefs more than religious affiliation (Pew Forum on Religion and Public Life 2008).

According to figures from 2007, there are 1.3 billion inhabitants in China of whom hundreds of millions engage in diverse religious beliefs and practices. There are five official religions recognized by the Chinese government. These are Buddhism, Taoism, Islam, Catholicism, and Protestantism. The Chinese government estimates that there are more than 100 million Buddhists worshipping in Buddhist temples (16,000) and monasteries with 200,000 Buddhist monks and nuns. Most Buddhists are ethnic Han Buddhists who practice Mahayana Buddhism. The government-sanctioned Taoist Association reports more than 25,000 Taoist priests and nuns, Taoist temples (1,500), and Taoist schools (2). There are hundreds of millions of citizens who practice traditional folk religions (worship of local gods, heroes, and ancestors) which are often blended with Taoism, Buddhism, or ethnic minority cultural practices (US Department of State 2007). In Taiwan, the Taoist population is relatively speaking larger than in mainland China. More than 80 percent of the Taiwanese people practice traditional Chinese folk religions (including also shamanism, animism, and ghost worship). Self-described spiritual practice is also popular. The sect movement of *Falun Gong* still holds its popularity, with approximately 2.1 million adherents, in spite of the Taiwanese government's oppression of the sect in 1999 (US Department of State 2007).

Even though Confucianism and Taoism lost their status as national religions, their ethical influence remains strong in East Asian countries, including Korea, Japan, and much of southeast Asia, with approximately 5 million adherents. Taoism is practiced in the US by approximately 30,000 followers and approximately 2,000 in Canada. Taoism has enriched European and Asian cultures by introducing teachings of the Taoist classic text of *Tao Te Ching*, and promoting a holistic lifestyle and health practice that includes Chinese diet, art, martial arts, Qi-gong, and Chinese medicine (Smith 1986: 119).

History

Early Chinese religion originated from centuries of village agricultural life beginning in the eleventh century BCE. From early times, the Chinese believed in the existence of multiple gods and spirits in nature, gods of heaven and earth, and evil spirits (called *kuei*). They practiced ancestor worship, religious sacrifice, and offerings. During the Shang dynasty (1500–1040 BCE), the polytheistic and animistic religious beliefs were unified into a concept of a supreme God (*Shang Ti*) who was above all others gods and spirits, controlling human destiny on earth according to human deeds. Later, during the Zhou dynasty (770–200 BCE), the concept *Tian* or heaven developed, which controlled the spirits of the dead and bestowed "the mandate of Heaven" on individuals and worthy rulers. Additionally, ancestor worship, grave burial, and oracle bones for divination were introduced as religious practices (Oldstone-Moore 2003: 204).

The patriarchal and hierarchical feudal system of the Shang and Chou Dynasties was challenged by external invasions and subsequent appearances of new societal classes. Warlords, merchants, and serfs replaced the existing aristocratic class system. The feudal world fell apart. In search of solutions to the social and political instability, many Chinese philosophical schools sprang forth (400–300 BCE). These philosophical schools proposed distinctive concepts in order to bring peace and social stability. Confucianism and Taoism were two prominent philosophical schools. Confucius (551–479 BCE) proposed a strong and centralized government based on moral principles. Taoism, based on the philosophy of Lao-Tzu, favored no government at all (Hopfe 2007: 169). During the Han dynasty (220 BCE–206 CE), the teachings of Confucius won the argument with the Chinese imperial bureaucratic system consolidated through civil service examinations based on the texts and teachings of Confucius. Temples were built to honor Confucius. This bureaucratic society ran the country with Confucian values until the collapse of the Han dynasty.

Taoism opposed the morality-oriented government. Built on the philosophical theories of Lao-Tzu (sixth century BCE) and Chuang-Tzu (fourth century BCE), Taoism claimed that people should follow the natural and eternal way of the universe, *Tao*, not human principles. Philosophical Taoism was influenced by two sect movements: the Yellow Turbans (184–215 CE) and the Way of the Celestial Masters, sometimes referred to as the Way of Five Bushels of Rice (200–300 CE). The Yellow Turbans worshipped a mother goddess, Xi-wang-mu, the "Queen Mother of the West," who was believed to grant immortal life to those who chant her name (Overmyer 1986: 27–31). The Way of the Celestial Masters was initiated by Chang Tao-ling (34–156 CE), the founder and first leader of organized Taoism, who spread it to the public by introducing healing practices such as exorcism. Celestial Masters were exposed to mystical experiences and alchemy. They gradually established a religious system that included various rituals and chanting. The two sects laid the foundation upon which Taoism would be consolidated into an organized religion (Unschuld 1985: 39).

The traditional religions – Confucianism and Taoism – were colored by Buddhism, which was introduced from India to China in the third century CE. Buddhism introduced a complex Indian cosmology and the concept of universal salvation. The collapse of the Han dynasty in 206 CE allowed people freedom to choose their own religion and religious practice. Buddhists' ability to contextualize their faith (600–700 CE) enabled them to spread their influence. In the process, they developed the new concept of Pure Land in the afterlife and a new method of meditation called *chan* (*zen* in Japan). Pure Land Buddhism attracted a wide range of people and met needs in uncertain times with its devotional practices and promise of rebirth in a future world. Chan Buddhism resonated with philosophical Taoism, sharing the quest for the true nature of reality. Taoists even incorporated Buddhist teachings and monastic lifestyles and encouraged celibacy in pursuing religious life by adopting a nunnery system (900–1000 CE). In spite of its efforts, Buddhism has always been identified as "a foreign religion" by the Chinese and suffered periods of persecutions under the Confucian majority (Oldstone-Moore 2003: 205–6).

After its decline, Confucianism was revived during the Song dynasty (960–1279 CE) and spread its influence beyond China into Korea, Vietnam, and Japan. This period is called "the second great wave of revival" in Confucianism (Berthrong 2003: 26). When China was reunified under the Chin Dynasty (1115–1234 CE), Confucian philosophy was thriving again, having developed into a new form that has come to be known as neo-Confucianism. Chu Hsi (1130–1200 CE), the founder of neo-Confucianism, developed a complex belief combining Confucian morality with Buddhist meditation. He claimed that all things, including human nature, have an ordering principle, *li*, which is the source to shape the vital material *ch'i*. Humans must cultivate themselves in order to understand the underlying principle of *li* (Overmyer 1986: 48–51).

Reliance on the impersonal principle (*li*) in neo-Confucianism, however, led many educated people to search for more personal and emotional gods and religious experience. Popular religious practices and activities such as shamanism, veneration of ancestors, divination, belief in ghosts and demons, and exorcisms began to rise again. This is known as the Chinese folk religion, which combined diverse aspects of major concerns of the three religious traditions, but without a systematic belief system. Popular folk religion dealt with the worldly and practical issues such as longevity, prosperity, domestic harmony, continuing the family line by bearing children, and protection from disaster. While Confucians rebuked popular religious practices, Buddhist and Taoist priests went close to the people by conducting various folk rituals (Overmyer 1986: 48–51).

Since then, Confucianism, Taoism, Buddhism, and folk religion have been blended together and practiced as Chinese religion. New religions (Islam, Christianity) were introduced to China during the Ch'ing dynasty (1644–1912 CE). Under the Cultural Revolution (1966–1976 CE), however, all religions in China were suppressed and violent actions were taken against religious practitioners. Folk religions, Confucian temples, and even Confucius' birthplace were destroyed; Taoists shrines, altars, tablets, and relics were purged. With the death of the communist leader Mao Zedang, the Chinese government reintroduced religious freedom and allowed religious activities, writings, and clergy – albeit subject to government sanctions. Centers for religious studies were reestablished in universities. The movement to restore Confucian teachings dating back to 1503 began to rise again. In Taiwan, on the other hand, popular Chinese folk religion and Taoism have long flourished with very few restrictions. On the whole, the four streams of the Chinese religion are thriving once again in Chinese society (Hopfe 2007: 177–87).

Beliefs and practices

General

The diverse and complex beliefs in Chinese religion are deeply rooted in ancient Chinese cosmology. The Chinese believed that *ch'i* was the vital substance that made up everything in the universe. *Ch'i* was thought to be manifested into *yin* and *yang* (the two complementary forces of the universe) and into five elements (metal, wood, water, fire, and earth) as the basic materials on the earth. Through *ch'i*, all things in the universe were co-related, interfused, and intermingled. There was interaction between heaven and earth, human beings and nature, and *yin* and *yang*. Ancient Chinese saw reality as constantly changing and transforming in the interaction between *yin* and *yang* and among the five elements consisting of wood, fire, earth, metal, and water. Thus, existence in the universe could not be just a well-ordered static condition but the perpetual activity of creating a harmonized unity. The concept of harmony is the center of Chinese thought and is the common theme of Confucianism and Taoism (Chan 1963: 244–5).

Confucianism centered on creating social harmony on the basis of virtues. Confucius (551–479 BCE) studied classics, rituals, poems, and legend in order to restore peace and order in society. He realized the importance of ethical principles that can be applied to everyone. There are basic virtues that Confucius promoted. These are *jen* (benevolence to humanity), *li* (rites, traditional ceremonies, and formal patterns of conduct), and *chun-tzu* (superior person). *Jen* served as an inner ethical commitment and responsibility of the rulers to create a good government for their people. Confucius taught in his classic *Analects* that the inward power of empathy and compassion for others is the basis of morality. This should be expressed in daily life through *li* (courtesy). For Confucius, *jen* and *li* were two golden ethical standards that should be expressed in the form of virtues through the five basic human relationships (Hopfe 2007: 181).

The five basic human relationships, according to Confucianism, are the foundation of a morally principled, well-ordered, and harmonious society. These relationships exist between the paradigmatic father and son in which father has to behave kindly to his son and the son respects the father in filial piety. The relationships extend to elder brother (gentility) and younger brother (humility); husband (righteous behavior) and wife (obedience); elders (consideration) and juniors (deference); and rulers (benevolence) and subjects (loyalty). Confucians believe that family relationship and the virtue of filial piety (*hsiao*) among the five basic human relationships is the foundation to bond the family and community, thereby ultimately harmonizing and transforming society and cosmos (Hopfe 2007: 181).

A Confucian virtue-based harmonious society can be achieved through education and self-cultivation. Self-cultivation is the process to become an authentic person who is honest to self and loyal to others. The individual can expand and deepen communal action for humanity through education and self-discipline. Confucius called the fully developed moral self "superior person" or "gentleman" (*chun-tzu*). The gentleman is a man of *jen*, a harmonized self, which is expressed in appropriate moral conduct or courtesy (*li*) in social relationships. *Jen* and *li* are manifested in loving one another, and practicing respect and courtesy toward one another. They are the inner moral core that motivates and guides a person to pursue the universal moral law of *Tao*, the foundation of the socio-political order of society. This is what Confucius calls respecting *t'ien-ming* (the mandate of heaven), which both the ruler and people must respect as the first principle. It is "the Way" (*Tao*) of heaven and the principle (*li*) of heaven or nature. Confucius' teaching of harmony claims that "human beings can make the Way (*Tao*) rather than the Way can make human beings great" (Chan 1963: 15–16).

On the contrary, Taoism views the universe as being operated by *Tao*, which they understand as the mysterious way of the universe. The tradition of philosophical Taoism dates back to Lao-Tzu (sixth century BCE), the legendary founder of Taoism. He served the imperial bureaucracy and promoted a laissez-faire theory of government. His *Tao Te Ching* is the classic text of Taoism, which is composed of a short text with only 5,000 words. Taoists believe that everything in the universe (human knowledge, achievements, education, and morality) is transient and temporary and will decay. Nothing is to be viewed more precious than life itself on earth, thus enriching and prolonging life should be a person's primary concern. The best way of enriching an individual's life is to live in perfect harmony with *Tao*, the source and origin of all life, which, as the first cause, existed even before *yin* and *yang*, and heaven and earth (Hopfe 2007: 172).

To follow the natural state of *Tao* requires a human being's non-intervention. The natural way of *Tao* itself is in perfect state and should be left alone. The individual has to take on a non-active, non-purposive state in order to access the *ch'i* (breath or life energy) of *Tao*, which is manifested as *yin* and *yang*, the two forces of nature. *Ch'i* forms and dissolves all things in the universe. Non-interference (*wu-wei*) is the best way that the individual can be tuned to and be harmonized with *Tao*, thereby accessing the maximum of *ch'i* for a healthy and long life, even achieving immortality. "Vitalizing Taoists" who utilized *ch'i* attempted to remove obstructions in the flow of *ch'i* and maximize it through breathing techniques and practicing immortality (a health and spiritual practice that aims at cultivating inner and outer self in order to achieve spiritual immortality). The practice of immortality was later reinforced by religious Taoists who claimed divine revelations for immortality and led temple worship services, rituals, exorcism, and healings for spiritual communities. Taoists pursue self-cultivation of *ch'i* and *yin-yang* balance in interaction with the harmonious relationship with the *Tao*. While Confucians pursue a harmonized self based on self-cultivated virtues or moral principles, Taoists pursue a harmonized self based on a simple, spontaneous (*tzu-jan*), and tranquil lifestyle (Smith 1986: 128–34).

Both Confucians and Taoists aim at conserving *te* (virtue) as the goal of self-transformation. For Confucius, this *te* is a perfect moral state, a manifestation of the universal moral law of *Tao* (Unschuld 1985: 60–2). Taoists view that *te* is a simple and weak way to let nature flow and take its own course. It is not a passive withdrawal from reality or government, but a practical strategy to oppose the controlling morality-based government at the time. Taoists view that self-transformation can take place by pursuing a natural lifestyle following and nourishing one's own human nature, *Tao*, as well as enjoying and returning to nature (Chan 1963: 136–7). Chuang-Tzu explained that he himself harmonizes all things in the universe and transcends the self beyond the control of the government. As disparate as they are in their approaches, Confucianism and Taoism are in common pursuit of harmony with *Tao* in their core. The Confucian balanced self is achieved through harmonious human relationships in social settings, while the Taoist balanced self is pursued in harmonious interaction with nature.

Pursuit of harmonious relationship with *Tao* in social settings and in the natural sphere was practiced through life events, religious activities, longevity, meditation, and seasonal occasions. Confucians' self-cultivating education was promoted through rituals that marked a series of life events. *Jiali*, a book of family rituals, describes the four basic Confucian rituals: capping (a coming of age ceremony for boys), wedding, funeral service, and ancestor worship (Yu 2002: 71–82). Ancestor worship was a central religious activity which carried from generation to generation reinforcing the core virtue of Confucianism: filial piety. Confucians believed that spirits of ancestors and of the dead have power to influence the lives of the descendants by either blessing or cursing them. Ancestor worship is a religious and communal activity in which human beings and divinities exchange a meal or offerings (Overmyer 1986: 24).

The Chinese medical ethical principle of "benevolence for all humanity" emphasizes the equality of all when providing treatment, regardless of gender, social status, age, etc. In the Chinese society, however, women's roles have been secondary to men in the domestic and public arena. Women developed a non-assertive self and sacrificed themselves for the sake of the harmony of the family. In medical practice, women have tended to hide their medical or family problems from outsiders in order not to bring shame or humiliation to the family. When the medical problems are related to contagious diseases, such as sexually transmitted diseases or HIV, women are more exposed to negative consequences (e.g., blame, physical violence, emotional torture, and abuse) from family and society. When men disclose sexually transmitted diseases, it is of less concern, even in cases of infection to other family members, due to the superior position that men hold in the family (Yang et al. 2006: 722). Thus, contrary to Confucian medical ethics, women today still face an unequal treatment in the patriarchal Chinese culture.

The Chinese have also taken seriously funeral rituals which were believed to send the deceased to a peaceful journey into the afterlife – a practice that shows a strong Buddhist influence. During the funeral ceremony, mourners throw dates on the coffin to ask the ancestors to bless their descendants with children. The Chinese believe strongly in the connection from the dead to the living and the past to the present. The harmonious relationship between them is considered to facilitate blessings for the living. The open coffin is placed in the main room of the house during the days of funeral rituals. During the services, food is offered to the spirit of the dead, and prayers are offered to gods for the deceased loved one's safe passage to the underworld. The appropriate gravesite for the deceased is often chosen through *feng-shui* (wind and water) to ensure a safe and peaceful place for the deceased and for the living to receive benevolence and blessings from ancestors. *Feng-shui* pursues the sacred power in the natural environment and a harmonious life within the natural order (Yang et al. 2006: 61–3). In recent years, it has become popular even in the West as a method to access prosperity and harmony in the home, workplace, and the business world (Oldstone-Moore 2003: 223).

A variety of meditation techniques have grown out of these early alchemy techniques. All three Chinese traditions – Confucianism, Taoism, Buddhism – practice meditation. Confucians practice "quiet sitting" in order to reflect on Confucian teachings or meditate on patterns of order (*li*) to strengthen the moral order of society. *Chan* (*zen*) meditative Buddhist groups practice the emptying of the egocentric mind and thoughts in a support group atmosphere. Taoists employ meditative techniques to enhance a new awareness of the cosmic power within the practitioner's body (Overmyer 1986: 77–9). Taoist alchemy masters teach people through meditation to help them internalize the spiritual forces of *ch'i* (life energy), *shen* (spiritual consciousness), and *Tao* (Kirkland 2002: 178). The pursuit of harmony between the mind and the body is the basis of all meditation techniques.

The blended aspects of the Chinese traditions are broadly celebrated through seasonal events as well. The Pure and Bright Festival (early April) is the occasion when the descendants visit the graves of the ancestors. The boat races and rice cakes of the Dragon Boat Festival (June) celebrate the highest *yang* power on earth and the beginning of the *yin* power. During the Dragon Boat Festival, Taoists still practice exorcism and drive out evil spirits thought to cause diseases or harm among people. Buddhism has influenced the All Soul's Day (late August) as an occasion to release the souls of ancestors or wandering spirits from the underworld (the place where the souls that have not been reborn reside) through offerings. Finally, during the autumn Harvest Festival and winter holidays, ancestors, hero gods, or patron saints are worshipped through thanksgiving (Hopfe 2007: 185–6).

Health and disease

To follow the natural rhythm of *Tao* is the central thought that has formed the health belief of the Chinese. *Tao* is manifested in dynamic changes of the *yin-yang* energies, allotment of *ch'i*, and interaction of the five elements of water, fire, wood, metal, and earth. According to Taoists, humans and nature are mutually interdependent. Humans have to conform to the natural rhythms of the universe in order to achieve health and longevity. Harmony between *yin* and *yang*, free flow of *ch'i*, and balance among the five elements are the three most important elements in understanding the Chinese concept of health and illness (Ni 1995: 17).

When there is harmony between *yin* and *yang* and among the five elements in the body, there is a natural flow of *ch'i*. The Chinese believed that *ch'i* is embedded in all existence, whether humans, trees, rocks, etc. *Ch'i* is part of the energy in the human body. As an allotment of *Tao*, *ch'i* is expressed in the *yin* and *yang* forces, balancing the interaction of the five elements (wood, fire, earth, metal, and water) that correspond with the human body, such as the heart (fire), the liver (wood), kidneys (wood), the pancreas (earth), and the lungs (metal). Human body parts interact with nature through *ch'i*. When a person is attuned to the natural flow of *ch'i* in nature, she or he may become healthy. If the *ch'i* flow in the body is blocked by such "evils" as weather conditions (cold, hot, wind, damp, etc.), *ch'i* deficiency or excess, or emotional stress, disharmony of the *yin* and *yang* energies occurs, leading to a break in the nourishing cycle among the five elements and resulting in diseases and death. Death is the state of complete separation between the *yin* and *yang* energies.

In the Chinese view, the human body is a holistic microcosm that embraces *ch'i*, *yin*, and *yang*, and the five elements in interaction with the macrocosm of nature. This health concept is not just limited to the physical aspect of the human body but also includes psychological and spiritual elements in interaction with nature and the environment. A holistic concept of health under the influence of *Tao* (*ch'i*, *yin*, and *yang*, and the five elements) is applied to diverse health practices among the Chinese. Chinese medicine, meditation, exercise, and nutrition therapy are common health practices. These practices when held in balance promote a natural lifestyle that helps incline a person to the natural rhythm of *Tao*, which contributes ultimately to enhanced health and longevity.

Common tools in the practice of Chinese medicine include acupuncture, herbal practice, nutrition therapy, and exercise. Acupuncture emphasizes that *ch'i* in the body is circulated via 12 meridians or channels to nourish the five major organs (liver, heart, spleen, lungs, and kidneys) and other parts of the body. When *ch'i* is obstructed, it creates imbalance between the *yin* and *yang* energies in patterns of either excess or deficiency, hot or cold, or interior or exterior to the body. Disharmony between the *yin* and *yang* energies causes abnormality and disease. Thus the goal of acupuncture treatment is to restore the balance of the *yin-yang* energy, hot and cold, exterior and interior, and deficiency and excess patterns in interaction with *Tao*. This *yin* and *yang* energy balance is believed to not only prevent diseases but also enhance the immune system (Bowman and Hui 2000: 1482).

Acupuncture is considered one of the most safe, effective, and low-cost healthcare modes, with few side effects. Apart from usual meridian-oriented acupuncture treatment, diverse forms and techniques of acupuncture treatments are practiced – such as ear, hand, and scalp acupunctures, electrical acupuncture, and acupuncture treatment based on different body constitutions (Maciocia 1989: 320–2). Aside from acupuncture, other traditional Chinese treatments include herb therapy, nutrition (food), moxibustion (heat therapy using mugwort herbs), cupping, and *gua-sha* therapy (scraping the skin) to enhance the *yin-yang* balance.

Health practices of the Chinese also include mind therapy or mind–body therapy. Meditation is a popular form of exercise to achieve a deeper state of self-awareness. This meditative process includes psychological, physiological, and spiritual disciplines in order to reach a higher state of consciousness and create a peaceful mind. Animating meditation or yoga promotes the inner self (Smith 1986: 130–31). Mind–body exercises are practiced in the form of martial arts both in China and elsewhere in the world, including the United States – such as *tai-chi-chuan* and *ch'i kung*. Many Chinese elderly engage in these arts early in the morning, combining breathing exercises with slow body movements. They also provide a social and environmental context where people get to know one another. Daily devotion to these arts strengthens the mind–body unit and promotes the circulation of *ch'i*. *Ch'i kung* is also a viable alternative exercise whenever there is a barrier to other forms of exercise – be it due to old age, physical disability, or slow physical rehabilitation. For stress-related diseases, it promotes physiological and psychological well-being in a relaxed, calm, and energized environment (Jouper et al. 2006: 949–57).

The Chinese worldview upholds a respect for life at its beginning and its end. Chinese medical ethics is greatly influenced by the core Confucian belief of benevolence toward all humanity. This universal ethical value is practiced in order to venerate and respect human life. Regardless of social class, family background, age, or sex, caregivers are called to love people and sustain and prolong life (Confucianism) over accepting death as a natural process (Taoism) (Jouper et al. 2006: 949–57).

Births – and male births in particular – are welcomed in Chinese society. Therefore, the Chinese cultural attitude toward abortion is generally negative, particularly in the case of male fetuses. The Confucian principle of filial piety encourages reproduction, especially of male offspring, as a responsibility to one's parents. The Confucian valuation of life is further strengthened by the Buddhist teaching of compassion and prohibition against killing any living beings. Thus, life is always viewed as precious and the taking of a life is something to be cautiously dealt with. At the same time, Chinese women are allowed to take initiative in making a decision on abortion when there is a high risk of hereditary or genetic disability (Baoqi and Macer 2005: 27).

Death and dying

The Chinese have understood death and dying as part of life. Both Taoism and Confucianism view that life comes from the mother, earth, and *yin* and returns to the father, heaven, and *yang*. Death and dying is simply a natural flow of life to return to its origin – *Tao*, where life starts. Even though Confucius' primary focus was on present life and human beings on earth, he dealt with the issues of death and spirits with sensitivity (Wei-ming 1986: 55–70). Ancestor worship and funeral rituals have strengthened the continuum of time between the dead and the living and between the past and the present. Taoists' understanding of death is similar to that of Confucians. Life and death are two complementary aspects of reality, the unchanging *Tao*; thus death is the change from being to non-being, from *yang* to *yin*. Death is considered to have equal value to life, thus death should not be feared. A contemporary Chinese thanatologist summarizes the understanding of the Chinese attitude toward life and death as *"zhong sheng an si,"* which means "respecting life seriously and accepting death peacefully." Confucians accept death with a willingness to preserve virtue and dignity, thus human beings should not be afraid of death. Humans can make a choice to die rather than making a non-virtuous effort to preserve life. Buddhists believe that death is a process of rebirth on the passage to nirvana (Tse et al. 2003: 339–43). When life on earth comes to its end, the Chinese perceive death as natural, even as an extension of life. The dying person feels safe and has a sense of belonging at home. Therefore, Chinese patients with terminal cancer usually wish to die in their own homes rather than in a hospital (Chen 2001: 270–3).

Withdrawing life support is still a difficult issue in China. When it is practiced in the settings of healthcare in the West, it should be handled with great sensitivity. It may be an offensive or reluctant issue for Chinese patients (Klessig 1992: 316–22). The centuries-long influence of traditional religious beliefs affects the issue of euthanasia. Buddhists view killing or shortening life as an evil act which will be punished in a subsequent life. The Chinese ethical principle of respect for life, influenced by Confucianism and Taoism, seeks to avoid advancing the process of death and dying. The Confucian ethical value of filial piety promotes keeping parents alive as long as possible. In spite of opposition to euthanasia among most lawyers in China, healthcare professionals and the public are paying more attention to the issue of quality of life for patients, thus passive euthanasia is being gradually accepted in China (Li and Chou 1997: 809, 243–8). The awareness of cultural differences in accepting and practicing death and dying will allow health practitioners to support end-of-life processes of Chinese patients with sensitivity.

Conclusion

Confucianism, Taoism, Buddhism, and popular folk religions have combined in the Chinese experience to form a diverse and complex system of traditions. Confucianism helped shape Chinese social roles and responsibilities. Taoism's mystical religio-philosophical tradition has pursued longevity in interaction with nature. Buddhism expanded and deepened traditional religious beliefs and spiritual practices. Popular folk religions embraced diverse aspects of each of these traditions and provided practical guidelines for daily life. Chinese religion is composed of practical and mystical traditions that have laid the foundation to create relational harmony between heaven and earth, between human beings and nature, and between the past and the present.

Table 7.1 Dos and don'ts

Dos	Don'ts
1 Grant the family as much influence and involvement as possible. 2 If need be, serve as a patient advocate if the possibility of family manipulation shows itself. 3 Recognize that medical decisions are not placed solely in the hands of the patient and may be solely in the hands of the family. 4 Know that more traditional Chinese may be reluctant to discuss advance directives. 5 Understand that most traditional Chinese will strongly desire to die at home.	1 Do not marginalize the family. 2 Do not be surprised at the presence of benevolent deception with terminally ill patients. 3 Do not bring up the topic of organ donation. 4 Do not speak openly about death as some believe that to do so may hasten death. 5 Do not hold on to prejudice against Traditional Chinese Medicine, which is widely practiced in Chinese-American communities. 6 Do not openly discuss mental disorder/disease and psychiatric services.

Case study

As the nurse educator for the surgical rehab unit where I worked, I had a reputation for having a lot of fun. My students and unit managers came to appreciate me filling that role. I especially highlighted ethical issues, mostly because no one else would touch it. I loved it and almost have a Master's degree in it now. The area I live in and the hospital I work for focuses a good deal of ethical attention to the issue of abortion, so it is often in my course material.

About a year ago, our hospital formed a "sister hospital" relationship with a hospital in China. The deal required multiple trips to China for educators from all over the hospital. I happily accepted an invitation to go as part of our clinical education team to focus on ethics, bioethics, and religion and ethics. Apparently, as Chinese culture becomes more open, their enforcement of atheism has softened and religion is becoming more important in the country. So they wanted me to talk about religion and ethics as part of my curriculum. Of course in the US religion and abortion is a huge issue and so I had thought I would include the topic of abortion in my course.

In the process of putting together my course, I was communicating routinely with the nurse educator on their end. I asked that she review my session goals and her response to abortion caught my attention. She informed me that, although she had a good deal of personal knowledge of religion, Christianity, and the topic of abortion in ethics and clinical ethics, she did not advise me to include abortion in my course material. In the past, China's "one child policy" had required enforcement such that forced abortions became routine. A very common reality for the women of China was that they were forced to have abortions whether or not they wanted one. Apparently, women of all faiths in China have a very high likelihood of experience with abortion. According to my educator partner on site in China, abortion was not a moral issue and did not make its way on to anyone's list of hospital or clinical ethics course material.

Questions for reflection

1   Is Christianity the only religion that argues about abortion as a moral issue? What do other religions teach on this topic?
2   If lots of religious people have undergone abortions in China, does that automatically take it off a list of ethical issues to be addressed in a hospital ethics course?
3   If the government forces someone to get an abortion and it is not a personal choice, does that remove the moral onus often associated with it?
4   What other moral issues emerge surrounding abortion in Chinese life and culture, if and when the issue of choice is taken off the table?

Glossary

Ch'i   Implies "breath of life" or "life energy," derived from Tao. In Chinese medicine, *ch'i* is the essence that maintains the functions of the body.

Chun-tzu   The name of the religious leaders who taught and practiced the five virtues of self-respect, generosity, sincerity, persistence, and benevolence to others.

Jen   Translated as "benevolence for all humanity." *Jen* in Confucianism is compared to the Golden Rule in Christianity: "Do not do to others what you would not like them to do to you" (Analects 15:23).

Li   Translated as "propriety, reverence, courtesy, and ritual." *Li* implies a person's right moral conduct that is expressed through ceremony, rites, and courtesy in the human relationships.

Tao   The origin of *Tao* is mysterious. It may be translated as the Path. But it is the Path that cannot be named or conceptualized. It encompasses everything. *Tao* is characterized as ultimate transcendent reality that guides the way of human life.

Wu-wei   Means literally "inaction." It implies "pure effectiveness" in Taoism and is often used to refer to a spontaneous act that emerges from harmony with the self and reality.

Yin and yang   The two complementary forces of the universe. *Yin* symbolizes night, dark, soft, cold, stillness, and feminine. *Yang* represents
day, bright, warm, movement, and masculine. All phenomena in the
universe are the expression of the interaction between *yin* and *yang*.
These two forces are opposite but mutually interacting and inter-
transforming.

Bibliography

Baoqi, S. and Macer, D. R. J. (2005) "A sense of autonomy is preserved under
Chinese reproductive policies," *New Genetics and Society*, vol. 24, no. 1: 15–29.

Berthrong, J. (2003) "Boston: The third wave of global Confucianism," *Journal of
Ecumenical Studies*, vol. 40, no. 1–2: 26.

Bowman, K. W. and Hui, E. C. (2000) "Bioethics for clinicians: 20, Chinese
bioethics," *Canadian Medical Association Journal*, vol. 163, no. 11: 1481–5.

Chan, W. (1963) *A Source Book in Chinese Philosophy*, New Jersey: Princeton
University Press.

Chen, Y. (2001) "Chinese values, health and nursing," *Journal of Advanced
Nursing*, vol. 36, no. 2: 270–3.

Hopfe, L. M. (2007) *Religions of the World*, revised by M. R. Woodward, 10th
edn, Upper Saddle River, NJ: Pearson/Prentice Hall.

Jouper, J., Hassmén, P., and Johansson, M. (2006) "*Qi-gong* exercise with concentration practice increases health," *American Journal of Chinese Medicine*, vol.
34, no. 6: 949–57.

Kirkland, R. (2002) "The history of Taoism: A new outline," *Journal of Chinese
Religions*, vol. 30: 178–83.

Klessig, J. (1992) "The effect of values and culture on life-support decisions," *The
Western Journal of Medicine*, vol. 157, no. 3: 316–22.

Li, S. and Chou, J. L. (1997) "Communication with the cancer patient in China,"
Annual of the New York Academy of Science, vol. 809: 243–8.

Maciocia, G. (1989) *A Comprehensive Text for Acupuncturists and Herbalists*,
Oxford: Churchill Livingstone.

Ni, M. (1995) "The manifestation of *yin* and *yang* from the macrocosm to the
microcosm," *The Yellow Emperor's Classic of Medicine: A New Translation of
the Neijing Suwen with Commentary*, Boston: Shambhala.

Oldstone-Moore, J. (2003) "Chinese traditions," in Coogan, M. D. (ed.) *World
Religions: The Illustrated Guide*, London: Duncan Baird Publishers.

Overmyer, D. L. (1986) *Religions of China: Religious Traditions of the World*, San
Francisco: HarperCollins.

Pew Forum on Religion and Public Life (2008) "Religion in China on the eve of
the 2008 Beijing Olympics." Available online at: http://pewforum.org/
docs/?DocID=301 (accessed December 10, 2008).

Schwartz, B. I. (1985) *The World of Thought in Ancient China*, Cambridge, MA:
Harvard University Press.

Smith, H. (1986) *The Illustrated World's Religions: A Guide to our Wisdom Traditions*, San Francisco: HarperCollins.

Tse, C. Y., Chong, A., and Fok, S. Y. (2003) "Breaking bad news: A Chinese perspective," *Palliative Medicine*, vol. 17, no. 4: 339–43, quoted from the original

Chinese edition by Zheng Xiaojiang (1994) *Philosophy of Death in the Chinese*, Taipei: Dong Da.

United States, Department of State (2007) *Report on International Religious Freedom*, The Bureau of Democracy, Human Rights, and Labor Report. Available online at: www.state.gov/j/drl/rls/irf/2007/ (accessed September 30, 2016).

Unschuld, P. U. (1985) *Medicine in China: A History of Ideas*, Los Angeles: University of California Press.

Wei-ming, T. (1986) "The Confucian tradition: A Confucian perspective on learning to be human," in Whaling, F. (ed.) *The World's Religious Traditions: Current Perspectives in Religious Studies*, New York: Crossroad.

Yang, H., Li, X., Stanton, B., Fang, X., Lin D., and Naar-King, S. (2006) "HIV-related knowledge, stigma, and willingness to disclose: A mediation analysis," *AIDS Care*, vol. 18, no. 7: 61–3.

Yu, Z. (2002) "Confucian education: A moral approach," *Religion East & West*, vol. 2: 71–82.

Suggested texts

Chan, W. (1963) *A Source Book in Chinese Philosophy*, New Jersey: Princeton University Press.

Fowler, J. and Fowler, M (2008) *Chinese Religions: Beliefs and Practices*, Sussex: Sussex Academic Press.

Overmyer, D. L. (1986) *Religions of China: Religious Traditions of the World*, San Francisco: HarperCollins.

Unschuld, P. U. (1985) *Medicine in China: A History of Ideas*, Los Angeles: University of California Press.

8 Sikhism

Arvind Mandair

> Ego is given to man as his disease. Disease affects all creatures that arise in the world except those who remain detached. Man is born in sickness, in sickness he wanders through birth after birth. Captive to disease he finds no rest, without the Guru sickness never stops.
>
> Adi Granth

Introduction

Sikhism refers to the way of life of those who call themselves Sikh, the way of life that embraces equality for all human beings and disapproves every form of discrimination on the basis of caste, race, and gender. Although the etymology of the word Sikh can be traced to the Sanskrit *sisya* or its Pali derivation *Sekkha*, the Punjabi term Sikh refers to the followers of Guru Nanak, his nine successors and their teachings embodied in the Guru Granth Sahib or the sacred scripture of the Sikhs.

Demographics

The Sikh population worldwide is estimated at 20 million. Of these, 17 million Sikhs reside in India, with 14 million of them living in the Punjab region – the traditional Sikh homeland. Of the two million or so Sikhs who live outside India, comprising what is known as the Sikh diaspora, the majority are dispersed in countries such as Great Britain, the United States, Canada, East Africa, Malaysia, and Australia.

It is estimated that 500,000 Sikhs live in the United States, with about 100,000 of them living in California. Yuba City, California (located 40 miles north of Sacramento) has the largest Sikh population in the country. There are 15,000 Sikhs living in and between Yuba City and Sacramento.

History

Sikhism originated in the Punjab region of Northwestern India during a time of Muslim–Hindu confrontation when a broadly aligned association of religious teachers known as the Sants were seeking to reconcile these two opposed cultural formations. The Sants expressed their teachings in vernacular poetry and distinguished the belief that salvation is to be based on inner experience rather than personalized incarnations. Although the teachings of Guru Nanak were broadly aligned with the Sants, his own mission emerged out of a direct experience of the divine initiated with the words *na koi Hindu, na koi Mussalman* (there is no Hindu, there is no Muslim) signaling a third way that was to become the *Nanak Panth* or the path of Nanak. The early community, which comprised those who chose to follow Nanak as their guru, was initially drawn largely from a Hindu background.

Nanak was born in 1469 (CE, and hereafter) in Talwandi, a village 40 miles from Lahore, and acclaimed by Muslims and Hindus alike as a future religious leader. Although he had received a formal education and held a post as a village accountant, Nanak's main preoccupation in his early life was with spiritual concerns and he preferred the company of saints and ascetics. Together with his closest associate, a Muslim bard named Mardana, Nanak organized regular nightly singing of devotional hymns, as well as going to bathe in a nearby river before daybreak. During one of these sessions, at age 30, Nanak underwent his first major mystical experience in which he received a calling to teach people a path of devotion to the divine Name. Shortly after this experience, Nanak embarked on a series of travels that took him eastwards to Banaras, Bengal, and Orissa, southward to Tamil Nadu and Sri Lanka, northward to Tibet, and finally westward to the Muslim regions going as far as Mecca, Medina, and Baghdad. In the final phase of his life at about the age of 50, Nanak founded a settlement at Kartarpur where he led a community of disciples instructing them in spiritual practice and study making *nam simaran* (remembrance of the Name) and *kirtan* (singing hymns of praise), regular features of devotion. At the same time he insisted that his disciples remain fully involved in worldly affairs by doing practical labor (Nanak himself tended his own crops) while maintaining a regular family life.

Shortly before his death in 1539, at age 70, Guru Nanak's appointment of a successor not only inaugurated a two-centuries-long politico-spiritual lineage with each successor taking on the title guru, but also marked a break with prior Sant practice of not appointing spiritual successors. During the next two centuries, the early Sikh Panth (community) underwent significant expansion and development into a defined and disciplined order, with different steps taking place under successive gurus. The second guru, Angad (1504–1552), collected Nanak's hymns, developed the alphabetic script called Gurmukhi (literally "from the guru's mouth") and institutionalized the *langar* or communal kitchen to feed disciples who came to visit Nanak's *dharamsalas*, or rest house. Guru Amardas (1497–1574), the third guru, encouraged the observance of separate Sikh shrines, pilgrimage traditions, and festivals, as well as instituting the *manji* system of supervising distant congregations. The fourth guru, Ramdas (1534–1581), founded a new center called Ramdaspur (later named Amritsar) where he supervised the excavation of the sacred pool that later became the central site of Sikh pilgrimage. Guru Ramdas appointed *masands* or deputies to represent the guru's authority in his more dispersed congregations.

Sikhism became more firmly established under the fifth guru, Arjan (1563–1606). However, the increasing success and expansion of the Sikhs in Punjab at this time led to confrontation with the Mughal imperial authority under the Emperor Jahangir. Guru Arjan was accused of supporting a rebellion led by Jahangir's son, Amir Khusro. Charges of sedition were followed by imprisonment and finally execution in Lahore in 1606. Guru Arjan's martyrdom led to increased militarization and overt political involvement under his son and successor, the sixth guru, Hargobind (1595–1644), symbolized by his donning of two swords, one representing spiritual authority (*miri*), the other representing political authority (*piri*). Maintaining a small but effective army, Hargobind consciously prepared the Sikhs to resist willful state oppression. Although confrontation receded during the tenure of his successor gurus, Har Rai and Har Krishan, they nevertheless maintained a similar style of leadership with a retinue of armed followers. It was the ninth guru, Tegh Bahadur (1621–1675), who again was forced to confront the increasingly restrictive policies of Jahangir's grandson, the Emperor Aurangzeb (1658–1707), which included enforcement of Islamic laws and taxes and the replacement of local Hindu temples by Muslim mosques. Guru Tegh Bahadur's active resistance against such policies, his public defense of Hindus' right to practice their religion freely, and his own refusal to accept Islam under pain of death led to his imprisonment and eventual execution in Chandni Chowk, one of Delhi's busiest markets, in 1675.

The Sikh Panth's involvement in political resistance came to a climax with the tenth guru, Gobind Singh (1666–1708). His best known contribution to the development of Sikhism was to redefine the very core of the Sikh Panth as a military-cum-spiritual order, the Khalsa (sovereign or free). According to tradition he called his followers to assemble for the Baisakhi festival in 1699 at Anandpur. There he called for five volunteers to pass a test of absolute loyalty. Those who passed the test, the so-called *panj piare* (Five Beloved Ones) were initiated into the new Khalsa order via a ceremonial rite called *khande ka pahul* (baptism of the double-edged sword), thus forming the nucleus of a sovereign, casteless community. Each member of the Khalsa order undertook to wear the five external symbols, or the five Ks (*kesh* – long, uncut hair; *kirpan* – short sword; *kangha* – comb; *kara* – steel bracelet; *kaccha* – breeches), to adhere to a formal code of conduct (*rahit*), and to relinquish family surnames with males assuming the name Singh (literally, lion) and females assuming the name Kaur (meaning princess), thereby removing sexual inequality whilst maintaining gender difference. The guru in turn received the same initiation from the *panj piare*, assuming the name Singh, signifying a merger of identities between the guru and disciple. Many thousands more accepted this initiation.

The creation of the Khalsa brought into existence a parallel, but two-tier system within the developing Sikh community. On the one hand, there were the Khalsa Sikhs, namely, those who took initiation into the Khalsa had effectively agreed to mark their bodies in a particular way – specifically by not allowing bodily hair to be trimmed, and in the case of Sikh males, of wearing a turban to cover the long, uncut hair. On the other hand were the so-called *Sahajdhari* Sikhs (slow adopters), those who in every other way lived by the teachings of the Sikh gurus but had not undertaken formal initiation into the order of the Khalsa. During the eighteenth and early nineteenth centuries, the relationship between Khalsa and Sahajdhari Sikhs was a relatively fluid one such that individual families could claim to have members belonging to both groupings. However, this distinction became more pronounced in the late nineteenth and early twentieth centuries and especially with the formulation of the modern Sikh code of conduct in 1954. This new code of conduct helped to establish Khalsa Sikhs as a more or less "orthodox" component of the Sikh community.

The advent of British colonial rule not only marks the entry of Sikhism into Western modernity, but also the emergence of several reform movements attempting to revive a sense of religious identity at a time when most such traditions were considered to be sects of Hinduism. By far the most influential Sikh reformist movement was the Singh Sabha founded in 1883 under aristocratic patronage. Through its political functionary, the Chief Khalsa Diwan (CKD), a body set up in 1902 to jointly conduct its affairs, the Singh Sabha movement achieved the most successful reinterpretation of a Sikhism adapted to modernity which has, until recently, exerted a hegemonic influence on Sikh self-consciousness. Their reformulation was based on the colonially inspired distinction between, on the one hand, a monotheistic-historical Sikhism centered on the authority of a clearly recognizable scripture and embodied by the Tat (authentic) Khalsa ideal, and on the other hand, a pantheistic ahistorical Hinduism. The leading Singh Sabha scholars redefined the doctrinal foundations of Sikhism in a way that would have been unimaginable only a few decades earlier. Under the banner of the Akali Dal, political successors to the Singh Sabha and the CKD, a campaign was launched in the early 1920s to wrest control of the Harimandar and other historical gurdwaras from the Mahants or traditional custodians, resulting in the Sikh Gurdwaras Act of 1925, which handed administration of these gurdwaras back to the Shiromani Gurdwara Parbandahk Committee (SGPC) – an elected body dominated by the Akali Dal party and which continues to dominate the religious and political affairs of the Sikh Panth. An important milestone for the SGPC was the publication of the *Sikh Rahit Maryada*, or the Sikh Code of Conduct, in 1953, which guaranteed greater uniformity of Sikh religious and ethical practices (Oberoi 1994).

Beliefs and practices

General

The distinctive nature of Sikhism can be traced to the thought of Guru Nanak which is embodied in his hymns that are part of the Adi Granth, amplified in the lives and works of his nine successors, and explained in the interpretations of Sikh scholars. For devout Sikhs, the most succinct articulation of Nanak's thought is encapsulated by the expression *ik oankar*, which appears at the very beginning of Nanak's *Japji Sahib* (the first and most authoritative hymn in the Adi Granth). This phrase is often translated as "One God Exists," though it is better translated as "The One Absolute Manifested Through Primal Word-Sound." According to Guru Nanak, the Absolute is non-dual (One). From the human standpoint, however, the Absolute is often perceived dualistically in terms of either/or distinctions such as *nirgun/sargun* (without qualities/with qualities; formless/form), or in terms of the difference between God and humans. But according to Guru Nanak, the Absolute cannot be conceptualized or obtained through rituals, through mere silencing of the mind, or by satisfying one's cravings. The Absolute can only be realized through experience. To realize the One, the ego-centered individual (*manmukh*) must be grounded in a state of existence that relinquishes the individuality of the self so that when the ego, or the self, is dropped off, the person (heart/mind/soul) emerges to merge with the Absolute, or the One. In this state, the person instinctively avoids relating to the One in terms of subject and object. Such a realized individual (*gurmukh*) no longer makes a conscious distinction between I and not-I, leaving an ecstatic and purely spontaneous form of existence (*sahaj*).

In Sikh tradition, the figure of the *gurmukh* and the spontaneous freedom associated with it are seen as an intensely creative form of existence that is "oriented toward the guru" and aligned with the divine order. The transition from duality to non-duality (or the transition from *manmukh* to *gurmukh*) is made possible through *naam* (the Name). In Sikh thought, *naam* is the medium through which the ego loses itself in human communication with others and experiences non-duality. In Nanak's hymns, *naam* is not a particular word or mantra, but is both comprised and written within the vibration of the cosmos. Being the link between mystic interiority and worldly action, *naam* is experienced by the *gurmukh* through the practice of *simaran* (constant remembrance or repetition of the Name), a form of meditation in which the One simultaneously becomes the focus of an individual's awareness and his motivation to perform righteous action. However, *naam* cannot be obtained voluntarily. Its attainment depends on grace or the favorable glance of the guru which leads to change in the individual from his birth nature to the spontaneous being of the *gurmukh*.

Thus, the guru in Sikhism takes on a role that goes well beyond what the word means in Hinduism where it is limited to a teacher. In Sikhism, the term guru includes this earlier meaning and goes beyond it to refer to the same divine light manifested in the ten historic gurus. Practically it serves to indicate the authority vested in the name Nanak. Just before the death of the tenth Nanak, Guru Gobind Singh, authority was jointly vested in the Adi Granth (hence, Guru Granth Sahib) leading to the doctrine of scripture or Word as guru (*shabad-guru*) and in the collective wisdom of the initiated community, the Khalsa, giving the doctrine of panth as guru (*guru-panth*). Underpinning all of these notions is the additional notion of guru as the divine principle itself. Therefore, a guru can simultaneously be a wise teacher, scripture, community, and the divine principle that under-girds the way of the Sikh tradition.

In matters of ethics, Sikhs turn for guidance primarily to sources such as the Adi Granth (or Guru Granth Sahib), and in addition, to secondary literature such as the compositions of Bhai Gurdas, the Dasam Granth, Janamsakhis, Rahitnamas, and to a modern document, the *Sikh Rahit Maryada* (Sikh Code of Conduct). The nature of the central Sikh scripture, the Guru Granth Sahib, is ideologically fluid in the sense that it does not allow readers to easily form absolute and concrete responses to issues that they are concerned with. This is partly because of the strongly poetic nature of the text and the fact that it resists the "God–Humanity–World" schema which everyone normally associates with religion. Instead, its main focus is the transformation of the ego. Not to annihilate the ego as such, but to reach a balance between ego and ego-loss, in order to attain a certain kind of personality or state of existing-in-the-world, or *gurmukh*. To the uninitiated reader, this lack of rigid ideology and imperative (such as "you *must* do such and such") can be disconcerting. But for Sikhs it frees the individual to think outside of all constraining ideologies and to think of self almost as an artist freed to create new values, rather than simply following a set of rules. This freedom is one that takes human beings beyond simple oppositions such as good versus evil, right versus wrong, violence versus spirituality.

Despite the conceptual fluidity of the Guru Granth Sahib, the representation of the text's central teaching underwent a major revision in the early twentieth century in the hands of a neo-colonial Sikh reformist movement, the Singh Sabha. This movement was essentially a response to the proselytizing activity of Christian missionaries and to the misrepresentation of Sikh philosophy by Indologists and conservative Hindu organizations such as the Arya Samaj. The resultant modification of Sikh teaching and practice can also be seen in the way they are represented in the West, primarily in English. What we read today as "Sikh ethics," "Sikh history," or "Sikh theology" are basically responses by modern Sikhism to a colonial demand for such categories, which are not native to the Sikh tradition. Thus in formulating ethical or religious responses to issues of health practice, one must be aware that there are differences between the approach that relies on the Guru Granth Sahib and Sikh gurus for guidance and one that utilizes modernist ideology and methodology such the Sikh Code of Conduct (*Sikh Rahit Maryada*).

Health and disease

Disease

Disease, according to its modern conception, is an unhealthy condition, an illness or sickness of the body and mind. Such a definition presupposes that the body has a normal condition which is health and wholeness. Health, in turn, has been defined by the World Health Organization as a "state of complete physical, mental and social well-being and not merely the absence of disease or infirmity," but is more narrowly conceived by many practicing physicians as the body's physical display of vital statistics determined by medical science (Singh 2008: 32–43).

While such definitions are perfectly acceptable to Sikh philosophy, they are also far too narrow. Their narrowness results, on the one hand, from having reduced the idea of health only to what can be seen, measured, and replicated according to scientific criteria, and on the other hand, from having determined health as opposed to disease. In the teachings of the Sikh gurus, however, health and disease are ontologically connected. This is because body and mind are considered to be part of a continuum rather than opposed. Health is, therefore, imaginary if only because it is temporary. The real state of our being is "dis-ease." In this sense, disease is not episodic but chronic. Dis-ease is a condition of existing in time and the world, but without being in tune with its ebbs and flows and without realizing its transitory nature. Therefore, loss of self and the collapse of the body are normative conditions.

In Sikh scripture, disease is not always "causally" linked to a bodily mis-function, but to the way in which human beings fundamentally exist in the world – namely, the state of ego. Disease occurs when a person asserts "I am myself" and turns this enunciation of the state of being into a defensive posture resistant to the flows of nature. Thus Guru Nanak says:

> Ego is given to man as his disease. Disease affects all creatures that arise in the world except those who remain detached. Man is born in sickness, in sickness he wanders through birth after birth. Captive to disease he finds no rest, without the Guru sickness never stops.
>
> (Adi Granth: 1140)

In a sense this may seem to suggest that disease is incurable, or that it is not ultimately important to cure disease since any cure will be temporary.

This means to perceive disease and the person who is marked with disease not as that terrifying other that must be stigmatized and isolated, but rather as something or someone who is already part of myself. Does this mean, then, that disease is simply illusory and that the pursuit of cure and of effective medicine is in vain?

On the contrary, based on the gurus' teachings on selfless giving and sacrificial care for others, Sikhs have been active in medical and philanthropic enterprises. They have also been very open to modern medical advances. The Sikh gurus, for example, vehemently rejected all manner of superstitious practices prevalent in South Asian culture, such as the belief that disease is caused by the "evil eye," black magic, or evil spirits. They also discarded the notion that disease is the result of divine punishment (Singh 2008: 35). Rather, the gurus built hospitals and sanctuaries in which they themselves worked to heal the sick, particularly those afflicted by leprosy and smallpox. Sikhs, both rich and poor, regularly donate money to build hospitals and schools in South Asia. Organ donation is a common trend amongst Sikhs and considered to be a good example of selfless giving. Such giving arises from the belief that the body is perishable and not needed in the cycle of rebirth. The real essence for Sikhs is the accumulation of memory traces that comprises one's soul. The final act of giving and helping others through organ donation is both consistent with and in the spirit of Sikh teachings.

While the medical and nursing professions are highly regarded within Sikh tradition, health practitioners should nevertheless be aware that attitudes amongst Sikhs may vary depending on the individual's level of education and social background. Also, many Sikhs are increasingly turning away from the industrial drug-based approach of modern medicine toward a more holistic view of disease. This is partly the result of a resurgence of interest in alternative modes of therapy. Reliance on homeopathic doctors is becoming increasingly common as patients become more aware of the negative side effects of modern chemical treatments. This resurgence has been aided by South Asian television programs which routinely teach yoga, Ayurvedic medicine, and other techniques to combat a large variety of ailments.

Dietary rules

Despite the fact that communal eating and the sharing of food has been and continues to be so central to the Sikh way of life, the current Sikh code of conduct (*Sikh Rahit Maryada*) has left the question of dietary rules unresolved or ambiguous at best. This is perhaps not surprising when we consider that the primary source of Sikh ethics, the Guru Granth Sahib, does not provide hard and fast rules concerning diet. Instead it offers more philosophical and pragmatic advice about avoiding or eating in moderation such foods that could potentially harm the body and mind.

Nevertheless, Sikh communities throughout the world have adopted a fairly consistent attitude toward certain kinds of food. For example, as a rule, no meat or intoxicants are served in Sikh gurdwaras (or temples), all of which have a communal kitchen attached to them. Foods prepared within the gurdwara have to use wholesome natural products, primarily milk, flour from wheat or corn, and vegetables. A variety of Punjabi tea is also served in many Western gurdwaras, but this is not the norm. Sikhs initiated into certain Khalsa orders are strictly vegetarian, with one or two exceptions. The Sikh Code of Conduct does not prohibit meat eating but it does state that animals should be slaughtered as humanely as possible with a single blow. Only beef is strictly avoided as most Sikhs come from a rural background. Since the cow, buffalo, and ox were central to the livelihoods of many rural Sikhs, these animals are treated with respect and never slaughtered for consumption.

Spouse, marriage, and family

Sikhs are strongly encouraged to adopt the life of a householder. Self-realization is best achieved as a member of a family and not through withdrawal from society to become a monk or a recluse. With the exception of the child-guru Harkrishan (who died at the age of nine), all of the Sikh gurus took spouses, had children, and lived lives that combined the roles of householder, warrior, and spiritual preceptor. However, the gurus also realized that this would be the most demanding way to live. It was much easier to run away from social issues, by renouncing family ties and becoming an ascetic. Nevertheless, Guru Nanak rejected renunciation and advised his followers to:

> Remain in towns and near the main high roads, but be alert. Do not covet your neighbor's possessions. Without the Name inner poise can't be attained nor can we still our cravings. The Guru has shown me that the real life of the city, the real life of the shops, is attained by achieving inner harmony. We must be traders in truth, moderate in our eating and sleeping. This is the true yoga.
>
> (Adi Granth: 939)

Echoing the strong emphasis on practicing spirituality within a worldly setting, the Sikh gurus gave women an exalted place within society. In a much quoted verse, Guru Nanak castigates medieval Indian society for looking down on women because they menstruated or bore children. Even more vehement was the guru's condemnation of *sati*, the self-immolation of women at the funeral pyres of their husbands:

> We are born from a woman, and in a woman we grow. We're engaged to and wed a woman. We take a woman as lifelong partner, and from

the woman comes family. If one woman dies we seek another. Without woman there is no social bond. So why denigrate woman when she gives birth to kings? Woman herself is born of woman, none comes into the world without her.

(Adi Granth: 473)

Other Sikh gurus further emphasized the status of women. Guru Amardas forbade women to veil their faces, while Guru Gobind Singh invited his spouse to become part of the ceremony for initiating Sikhs into the order of the Khalsa. In keeping with this, monogamy is therefore the preferred and predominant model. Widow remarriage is a relatively prevalent occurrence in contemporary Sikh society, although many other Sikh women choose not to remarry and remain single.

Sikhism encourages and generally follows a heteronormative model of marriage as a way to lead a wholesome life with a full expression of one's emotional, psychological, and biological impulses. However, because the joint or extended family is still the prevalent norm within North Indian society and even in the Western Sikh diaspora, marriage is not a private affair between two individuals. Rather it involves the joining of two families who become connected through the individuals. The concept of marriage in Sikhism is not based on a social contract but aims at the fusion of two souls into one. It is therefore analogous to the union of humankind with the divine, which is also the goal of Sikh spirituality. In this union humans are the lover (hence female) while the divine is the beloved (hence male). Marriage is the institution where spirituality is consummated: "They are not man and wife who have physical contact only. Only they are truly married who have one spirit in two bodies" (Adi Granth: 788). Physical consummation is therefore to be considered a necessary step toward a broader goal of awakening spiritual desire and longing for detachment within the very institution which joins two individuals. Such attachment, which is to be attained while being attached to another, is likened to the "blissful state" in which the mind attains union with the beloved.

Gender and sexuality

The representation of Sikhs in the Western media – bearded and turbaned men carrying swords and cases of female infanticide – gives the impression that Sikh society is patriarchal and misogynistic. Closer scrutiny suggests, however, that the role and status of women are more diverse and influential than portrayed in the media. Women have the same access to religious teachings and practices as men, and the transmission of basic spiritual and moral precepts to the next generation usually begins with women in their role as mothers. Though rarely acknowledged, the teachings of the Sikh gurus suggest that women have an innately greater spiritual potential than men. This is partly because the central obstacle in spiritual attainment is not simply the ego but the conflation of the ego, which is thought to be a typical attribute of maleness. This attribute hinders one's ability to tap the reservoir of emotions and moods necessary for achieving a balanced state of mind. Moreover, the nature and concept of God in the teachings of the Sikh gurus is not necessarily male. Divinity has equally feminine attributes.

Historically, women have risen to the highest positions in Sikh society. The tenth guru's spouse, Mata Sundari, not only played a key role in the creation of a new spiritual-cum-military order (the Khalsa), but after the guru's death led the Sikh community in spiritual and political matters, far longer than any male Sikh guru. Other women such as Rani Jindan (the spouse of the Sikh ruler Maharajah Ranjit Singh) wielded enormous power in the Sikh kingdom prior to British rule. In recent years, Bibi Jagir Kaur was elected the jathedar of the Akal Takht, the highest ecclesiastical position in Sikhism. All this has been possible because there are no scriptural or theological restrictions placed on women from having access to education or social, political, or spiritual ascendancy. Factors that prevent women from public endeavors have been due to the patriarchal culture of North Indian society.

Homosexuality

According to the value system of modern Sikhism as prescribed by the Sikh Code of Conduct (1954), Sikhs are expected to live in a family environment in order to properly nurture their children. Most Sikhs interpret the family structure to be based on a heteronormative model of sexuality. Many Sikhs have interpreted this to mean that homosexuality cannot result in procreation and is therefore unnatural. However, such a judgment bears a strongly Christian and especially Catholic imprint, which believes in natural law: "what is natural is what is moral." This can be seen in recent statements by Sikh religious leaders who not only openly condemned homosexuality as unnatural but seemed to justify their stance by reference to "other major world religions."

As a result of these strictures, many Sikhs with homosexual orientation have tried to enforce upon themselves "normalization" of their sexuality by convincing themselves that what they experience is merely lust and by marrying a member of the opposite sex and producing children. Such a process of forcing homosexuals to "go underground," as it were, has led to a belief among many Sikhs that there are no homosexual Sikhs. This belief can, in turn, cause distress to those Sikhs who happen to find themselves attracted to members of the same sex.

However, a closer look at the primary source of Sikh ethics, the Guru Granth Sahib, shows that while the question of homosexuality has not been explicitly discussed, there is no justification whatsoever for castigating and banning homosexuality. Moreover, South Asian culture has been traditionally tolerant toward the question of homosexuality, seeing it as one of the manifestations of ecstatic and erotic mysticism. Trans-sexuality and gender crossing is a well-known aspect of mystical enunciation, particularly in those movements influenced by bhakti (the path of devotion) and Sufism (mystical tradition in Islam). Many liberal Sikhs have called for new ways of interpreting Sikh scripture on the question of gender and sexuality which give greater credence to the trans-gendered "standpoint" of devotional love that is central to the Sikh gurus' teachings. Recent research suggests that such new interpretations are likely to complicate the issue considerably as the Sikh gurus' writings on love and eroticism may challenge the modern understandings of sexuality.

Abortion

The Sikh scriptures, the modern Sikh Code of Conduct, and related historical sources are silent about the question of abortion. As a result, individual Sikhs and Sikh communities in Punjab and in the Western diaspora have had to work out relevant responses based on their interpretation of the teachings of the Sikh gurus or by resorting to existing Punjabi cultural norms and shared traditions.

The Sikh scriptures do address important questions about the cycle of life and death that inform one's decision on abortion. It teaches that there is no absolute beginning or end to life, but that life continues beyond death in the form of a new birth. Thus, Sikhs who take the implications of this teaching seriously tend to believe that the moment of conception represents the rebirth of a fully developed person who has lived in previous lifetimes. To terminate a birth through abortion, then, would be tantamount to refusing a soul entry into a particular body and sending it back into the cycle of births and deaths – a choice that is not for human beings to make.

However, such a view is increasingly recognized by Sikhs today as idealistic and unable to provide suitable answers to instances when the mother's physical or psychological health is threatened, when there are problems with the fetus' health, or when the mother simply wishes to abort the fetus. Taking note of the fact that the vast majority of scriptural teachings do not directly address the issue of abortion, Sikhs influenced by the modern reformist tradition tend to interpret the gurus' teachings in a more pragmatic fashion. This pragmatism itself is grounded in the gurus' recognition of the mystery of life and death:

> None is informed, my trader friend, when death will come to send them off. When death comes to send them off is known to the Lord and no one else. Your family's lamentation is false, for the dead one is no longer their kin. What you get in the end is only that on which you fastened so much love.
>
> (Adi Granth: 74)

Consequently, neither modern Sikh society nor its religious authorities are concerned with laying down a rigid rule on abortion. But if there is a stricture regarding abortion which would be binding on all Sikhs, it would be that abortion should not be linked to any kind of personal gain, economic or otherwise, nor driven by selfish motives or by the five traditional vices of lust, anger, covetousness, attachment, and pride. Nonetheless, doctrinal ambiguity has had one significant negative social consequence in Sikh society – that of the continuing prevalence of female feticide (Coward and Sandhu 2000: 1167). This stems from a general bias in favor of males over females, which reflects Indian society's view of women, due to the dowry system, as economic liabilities. Elective abortion for this reason has been noted even among Sikh communities in North America. Though not an uncommon practice, this type of abortion would be considered acceptable for most Sikhs.

Contraception and reproductive technologies

For Sikhs there are a number of interlinked issues to consider with regard to contraception and reproductive technologies. How is life defined, particularly in Sikh scripture? If one could define life as such, at what point does life actually begin in the reproductive timetable? And is there a moral difference between not starting a life (contraception) and ending one (abortion)? As we have seen, although the scriptures are non-committal on this topic, there are hints that the definition of life is relatively fluid and would incorporate a continuum that includes non-sentient and sentient forms. According to the writings of the Sikh gurus, a properly moral issue can only arise when a new life becomes sentient. Even though sentience includes both unconscious and conscious states of existence, the crucial point of origin may not necessarily be the physical joining of sperm and ovum, but a later stage when the fetus becomes sentient. The difficulty of pinning this process down might explain why Sikhs are not acutely concerned about contraception except insofar as it becomes an act that results from and leads to one or more of the five vices. In addition, it is also helpful to remember that women in rural India have long used alternative techniques and traditional remedies to prevent conception and carry out abortions. Thus, contraception and abortion are not linked strongly to religious concerns as they may be in other cultures.

Given the strong emphasis in Sikhism on the family, the use of research and technology is generally considered an asset. With the Sikh Code of Conduct being generally silent on the issue of technology, Sikhs are likely to welcome new technologies such as *in vitro* fertilization. Although issues such as genetic engineering have not been routinely discussed in the community, given the non-dogmatic nature of the Guru Granth Sahib, Sikhs are unlikely to be opposed to such research given its potential to predict and eradicate cases of chronic disease such as Parkinson's disease, multiple sclerosis, Down's syndrome, and various types of cancer. Nevertheless, the current prevalence of female feticide in many Sikh and Punjabi households highlights the way in which reproductive technologies, such as those that enable parents to predict the sex of the fetus, can be used for purposes of questionable ethics.

Death and dying

Death is a powerful and abiding theme in the teachings of the Sikh gurus and more broadly within South Asian spirituality. Despite saying much about the fact and phenomenon of death, the Sikh gurus also acknowledge that death is and will remain a constant mystery, an irresolvable contradiction, not the least because death is intrinsically connected to life and existence rather than being opposed to it. Death and life are often mentioned and discussed in the same verse and often in the same line. In this sense the Sikh gurus perceive death differently from modern science, which defines death as the end of life caused by stoppage of the means of sustenance to body cells. In Sikh teachings, death underlies one's existence from the very start of life. As Guru Nanak says, "we entered this world with death written as our fate" (Adi Granth: 1126).

One of the key terms used for death is *kal*, which has a dual signification, connoting death as well as time. Both are philosophically and psychologically intertwined. *Kal* is often denoted as *jam kal* (Jama being the Vedic god of death). To the person who refuses to confront the true nature of time as here and now, the gurus project the intolerable face of time as one's own mortality. Through this depiction one is existentially confronted with the presence of death here and now. While ordinarily people lament the passing of time, grieving for things lost, and suffering when attachments are broken, the guru teaches that attachment and suffering result only from our habitual obstruction of the natural flow of time. By accepting time's impermanence as our own essence and seeing every attempt to control it as ultimately illusory, the individual can be released from suffering even while still living and thereby attain union with the divine. This is referred to as learning to die while still living (Adi Granth: 935).

Death is therefore not only the privilege of those who live life positively. It also marks the moment of union with the divine and the passage to the next birth. As such, it is not an occasion for grief. The desires, thoughts, and actions in any particular lifetime leave their traces in the memory of an individual. These traces influence the circumstances and predispositions experienced in future lives.

This non-linear, non-attached perspective on life and death sustains the practical way in which Sikhs deal with death. Since the body is useless after death, Sikhs practice cremation. Burial at sea is also permitted. After cremation, the ashes may be buried but normally the remains are dispersed into the nearest river. The cremation ceremony is a family occasion. The body is washed and clothed by members of the family who take care to ensure that it carries the symbols of the faith (*panj kakkar*, or the five Ks). The body is then taken to a cremation ground in India, or if the funeral happens to take place outside India, to a funeral home. During the journey, the mourners will sing hymns from Sikh scripture. During the cremation itself, the evening hymn is sung and the ceremony concludes with a prayer. On returning to the home of the deceased, the mourners begin a complete reading of the Guru Granth Sahib. Once the reading is completed over a period of 48 hours, the mourners will receive *karah parshad*, a sacramental food. The sharing of this food symbolizes the continuity of life in the midst of death.

Sikhs believe that human birth is a precious gift, an opportunity with which to harness the body's potential for adoring *naam* and serving others. Life is a field upon which the self can properly experience the twin registers of *sukh* (pleasure/enjoyment/happiness) and *dukh* (pain or suffering) as thoroughly intertwined. Although one's existence may be imbued with pain, Sikh teachings emphasize that one should not reject pain by labeling it bad, but rather accept it with the same demeanor that one accepts pleasure. From such a perspective, many Sikhs argue that taking one's own life is ethically wrong because the impulse to annihilate oneself emanates primarily and paradoxically from deep-seated self-attachment, the desire to cling to one's own life as if it were one's own to begin with. Moreover, suicide far from solving anything creates more pain for those left behind.

The case of euthanasia is more complex, however. To begin with, it is necessary to differentiate between active and passive euthanasia. Whereas active euthanasia implies the intentional hastening of death by a deliberate act, passive euthanasia can refer to the intentional hastening of death through a deliberate omission or withdrawal of things that might otherwise sustain life. Furthermore, euthanasia can be carried out against the wishes of the patient or actually be requested by the patient and undertaken by a third party such as a doctor. The modern and conventional Sikh response to euthanasia is to say that the decision to kill or ascribe death to a person in pain or undergoing other forms of suffering is based on delusion. The causal root of delusion can be traced to one or another of the five vices spoken of in Sikh scripture (Singh 1983: 31). In such cases, as the argument goes, the dying person and/or the person assisting the dying person should use the process of dying as an opportunity to reflect on the nature of self-attachment and other psychological charges associated with the five vices. The idea here is that as long as there is life, there is always hope. Sikhs contemplating euthanasia are encouraged to look at the whole of life and try to make the appropriate distinctions between ending life and not artificially prolonging a terminal state. For those who contemplate assisting the death of another, the emphasis of this argument is to provide greater care and service for others who are less fortunate.

While this theory works perfectly well in the cases where the motive for hastening death is physical suffering, complications can arise when we take into account other potential motives for hastening death. There are several historically important cases of Sikhs refusing to live in order to serve a noble cause, such as individuals who hasten their own death in order to save others. Two of the Sikh gurus (Arjan and Tegh Bahadur) willingly chose to be tortured and die rather than prolong their own lives and in so doing condemn their fellow men and women to subservience and misery. Their deaths had a powerful emancipatory force on the community. There are numerous other such examples in early and modern Sikh history. Of course, such death is normally classified as martyrdom, and not as euthanasia. But how distinct, philosophically and spiritually, is the concept of martyrdom from other types of death, especially when the idea of a good or proper death is so strong in Sikh scripture? Health practitioners may need to be aware, on the one hand, of the psychological motivations for an individual desire to hasten death, and on the other, of the deeply spiritual and often ambivalent nature of Sikh teachings on death.

Conclusion

Sikhism preaches the message of the One True God and the path leading to oneness with God through devotion, meditation, and elimination of one's ego. Sikhs' way of living also includes living a righteous life through promoting equality, resisting discrimination, and avoiding superstition. Religion is central to the practice of health and wellness since health is not merely defined by physical functionality but alignment with the ultimate goal in life, the path to the One True God, and disease therefore is understood as a state of dis-ease due to the attachment with the ego. From this

Table 8.1 Dos and don'ts

Dos	Don'ts
1 Be sensitive to same-gender care. 2 Respect modesty and privacy in patient care. 3 Respect personal space by limiting physical contact. 4 Be sensitive to the religious symbols of the Five Ks: uncut hair (*kesh*), a wooden comb (*kangha*), a steel bracelet (*kara*), underwear (*kachhehra*), and a ceremonial sword (*kirpan*). 5 Consult Sikh religious leaders/family in dealing with ethical issues. 6 Allow family to follow tradition when preparing dead body for the funeral.	1 Do not interrupt patients during prayer. 2 Do not remove hair from any part of the patient's body without consulting. 3 Do not insist on using only hospital gowns for Sikh women. 4 Do not offer meat used in religious sacrificial ceremonies or Halal meat to Sikh patients.

perspective, Sikhism sees medical advancement as an instrument for compassion that is in accord with Sikhs' belief in living a righteous life. Hence, within a clinical context, understanding and being intentional about religious beliefs and practices can greatly benefit Sikh patients in their recovery.

Case study

The genetics counseling clinic where I work is in a large, multi-cultural metropolitan area on the East coast. Despite the routine exposure to perspectives on decision making that baffled me on a personal level, the couple sitting across from me pushed me along paths I had not yet traveled. I had met them one year ago and helped them navigate issues they were having in the process of basic family planning. They wanted to have a baby and everything seemed fine.

Even prior to the attempt to get pregnant we discussed genetic testing methods that would work after conception to have some sense of the health of the child. After talking through the various methods and timing for such testing, they decided to use amniocentesis at 18 weeks pregnancy. We met after the results came back.

Everything was fine with the baby; a 21-week girl appearing completely normal in all of the analysis. So, I was more than a bit confused and thrown off when, after only a brief glance at each other, the husband said they would like me to refer them to a physician who could provide an abortion. I stumbled over my words, not so much about the idea of abortion, but that it seemed so dramatically against the flow of my clinical work with them over the past year or so. They did not lack any clarity, however, as they went on to tell me that they wanted a son and not a girl.

When I pushed further into the conversation, it was clear to me that there was a complex family dynamic going on behind the scenes; beyond the conversations I had been having with them. His family had recently moved to the US from Punjab and her family had been here for much longer. Both families and the two of them followed the Sikh religion, something I did not know much about. She herself was born in the States and two of her four siblings had sons already. In listening to her, it seemed the family pressure on her to have sons was, therefore, much less intense than in his family.

His family, according to what he shared with me, was another story altogether. He was the oldest of four children. Theirs would be the first grandchild for his side of the family and that was putting a lot more pressure on them than I could imagine. Indeed, his mother and father were waiting for them in the hospital café upstairs; anxious to hear whether or not their baby was a boy.

Questions for reflection

1   All the while talking with them about their quandary, I was thinking about my own personal sense of how to relate to their request. I did not appreciate their request and I certainly strongly disagreed with their cultural bias against girls. What should I say to them?
2   How much of my personal response should I include or should I just give them some information and stay out of it?

Glossary

Adi Granth   Translated as "the first" and refers to the early compilation of Sikh scriptures by the fifth Guru.

Gurdwara   Gurdwara is translated as "the door/path to the Guru" and refers to the Sikh temple.

Gurmukh   The idea behind *Gurmukh* is to follow the teachings of the Guru instead of giving in to one's inclination and desire.

Guru Granth Sahib   This body of literature is the Sikh's holy scripture and is regarded as the final authority for all Sikhs.

Khalsa   Khalsa means "pure" and refers to Sikhs who have been baptized or initiated through a special ceremony.

Sikh Rahit Maryada   The code of conduct incumbent upon all Sikh faithful.

The five vices   The five vices that beset human behavior are Kam (lust), *Krodh* (rage), *Lobh* (greed), *Moh* (attachment), and *Ahankar* (ego).

The five virtues   The five virtues taught by Sikh Gurus are *Sat* (truth), *Daya* (compassion), *Santokh* (contentment), *Nimrata* (humility), and *Pyare* (love).

Bibliography

Coward, H. and Sandhu, T. (2000) "Bioethics for clinicians: Hinduism and Sikhism," *Canadian Medical Association Journal*, vol. 163, no. 9: 1167–1170.
Oberoi, H. (1994) *The Construction of Religious Boundaries: Culture, Identity and Diversity in the Sikh Tradition*, New Delhi: Oxford University Press.
Singh, A. (1983) *Ethics of Sikhism*, Patiala: Punjabi University Press.
Singh, K. (2008) "The Sikh spiritual model of counseling," *Spirituality and Health International*, vol. 9: 32–43.

Suggested texts

AjitSingh, C. (2002) *The Wisdom of Sikhism (One World of Wisdom)*, Oxford: One World Publications.

Grewal, J. S. (1990) *The Sikhs of the Punjab*, New Delhi: Cambridge University Press.

Mandair, A. S. and Shackle, C. (2005) *Teachings of the Sikh Gurus: Selections from the Sikh Scriptures*, London: Routledge.

Nesbitt, E. (2005) *Sikhism: A Very Short Introduction*, New York: Oxford University Press.

9 Islam

Hamid Mavani

In the name of Allah, most benevolent, ever-merciful.
All praise be to Allah, Lord of all the worlds,
Most beneficent, every-merciful. King of the Day of Judgment.
You alone we worship, and to You alone turn for help.
Guide us (O Lord) to the path that is straight, the path of those You have
 blessed,
Not of those who have earned Your anger, nor those who have gone
 astray.

Qur'an, Surah 1

The Prophet said, "Give food to the hungry, pay a visit to the sick and
release (set free) the one in captivity (by paying his ransom)."

Hadith (Sahih Bukhari)

Introduction

Unless you keep yourself entirely isolated from the news in the United
States, you have been deluged in recent years with a plethora of articles
and images of Muslims and the Islamic religion. Impossible to miss was
the attack of September 11, 2001, on the Pentagon and the Twin
Towers of New York City by radical terrorists who referred to themselves as Muslims. Hopefully, you have Muslim friends or neighbors so
that you can appropriately balance what you are hearing and reading
about in the news and what you know by way of acquaintance and
neighborly familiarity. American culture is often referred to as Judeo-
Christian, leaving out the third of the monotheistic Abrahamic faiths:
Islam. American culture is more properly understood as Abrahamic and
not simply Judeo-Christian. In other words, Muslims and the religion of
Islam have had a great deal to do with the shaping of Judeo-Christian
cultures of Western civilization whether or not textbooks make note of
this fact.

Please do not allow the skewed portrayal of Muslims and the religion of
Islam found in the popular media to set the tone of your interaction with
Muslims – either personally or professionally. You will find, as you engage

Muslim patients and associates, many points of commonality with your own sense of tradition and faith.

Demographics

There are no precise and statistically sound demographic data available on Muslim Americans primarily because asking questions pertaining to one's religious affiliation is prohibited by the US Census Bureau and the United States Citizenship and Immigration Services. However, there is a general agreement that the Muslim numerical strength in America is a growing phenomenon with membership in important segments of society. Estimates range from two to eight million based on extrapolations.

There is a consensus that the three dominant groups are South and Southeast Asians, Arabs, and African American Muslims, with a group from the Hispanic and Caucasian communities that are converting to Islam. The American Muslim Council estimated in 1992 that the major groups are African Americans (42 percent), South Asians (24.4 percent), and Arabs (12.4 percent), along with Africans (5.2 percent), Iranians (3.6 percent), Southeast Asians (2 percent), and American Whites (1.6 percent) (Leonard 2003: 4). Another study conducted in 1999 by the Center for American Muslim Research Information estimated that Arabs account for 33 percent, African Americans for 30 percent, and South Asians for 29 percent of the Muslim American population (Leonard 2003: 4). All ethnic groups have their unique expressions and understanding of Islam. By and large, in contrast to the Muslims in Europe, they have been successful at integrating into the American society and face minimal tension in adopting American values and attitudes. However, about half of the Muslim respondents in the 2007 Pew Research Center survey identified themselves as Muslims first and then as Americans. When a similar question was posed to Christian Americans, about 42 percent considered themselves as Christians first (Pew Research Center 2007: 37).

Pew Research Center's August 2011 study estimated that the total Muslim population in the United States is 2.35 million, out of which 1.8 million are adults over the age of 18. Sixty-three percent are immigrant Muslims who have migrated for a variety of reasons from about 68 countries, and 37 percent are born in the United States. Sunni Islam, which is the dominant stream within the religion of Islam, comprises about 65 percent, and the minority, Shi'a Islam, consists of about 11 percent of the total Muslim American population (Nekola 2011). Whatever the numerical strength of the Muslim community, it is now a well-established fact that Islam is an important feature of North American religious milieu and is the fastest-growing religion in the United States.

The Muslim community in America comprises a mosaic of diverse ethnic and cultural groups that have embraced a variety of worldviews depending on its reading of Islam's two foundational sources: the Qur'an and the Sunnah. For Sunni Islam, the Sunnah is the record of the words and deeds of Prophet Muhammad, while for Shi'a Islam it consists of the words and deeds of the Prophet and his designated successors. There is unanimity among Muslims that the Qur'an is the timeless and inerrant Divine Word that was revealed to Prophet Muhammad over a period of 23 years, suggesting that it was intimately related to the life of the society of Arabia in the seventh century CE. The Qur'an remains the foundation of Muslim lands and their constitutions, and accordingly the precepts, moral imperatives, and spiritual values of the Qur'an become the norms for the Muslim community everywhere. The textual Qur'an is complemented by the exemplary figure of Muhammad, whose statements, actions, and tacit approval found in the Sunnah elucidate the Qur'an. Thus, the Sunnah constitutes the second major source in the formulation of Islamic law. Muslim jurists employ these two sources and other methodological tools and devices such as analogy, rational analysis, consensus, and consideration for public welfare to provide rulings and guidelines on temporal and religious aspects of the life of the Muslim. Accordingly, all acts are categorized by the jurists under a fivefold scheme of classification and given a value ranging from mandatory to the prohibited. The five values are: obligatory (*wajib*), recommended (*mandub*), permissible or neutral (*mubah*), reprehensible or discouraged (*makruh*), and prohibited (*haram*).

History

The journey of Muslims to America can be viewed in five stages: (1) they came as explorers and guides; (2) they came fleeing the persecution of Spain in the sixteenth and seventeenth centuries; (3) they came as a result of the Barbary Coast Wars and the slave trade on the coasts of West Africa; (4) they immigrated in the mid- to late 1800s primarily from Lebanon and Syria; and (5) they came in waves after the liberalization of the US Immigration and Naturalization Acts of 1952 and 1965, which removed the preferential treatment that was accorded to European immigrants.

There is a large percentage of today's African American population that can trace its heritage directly back to the slaves of West Africa and the survivors of the North African Wars. Among those who were captured were Muslims who were literate, fluent in Arabic, articulate, and determined to retain the rich heritage of their ancestral lineages. Muslims of African descent are not a new phenomenon on the American continent. The root sources of Islam in America, the questions of race, and the development of African American Muslim identity are the natural outgrowth of these early religious pioneers and their struggle for survival, freedom, equality, and faith.

In this context, Islam, as a different and foreign religion and a "color-blind" community that seeks to transcend ethnicity and culture, had a great appeal to the Nation of Islam and other African American groups.

Islam provided them with a new form for self-identification and liberation from American culture and history. The Ahmadiyya movement, which is regarded as a heretical group by most Muslims, was the primary avenue through which the African Americans received knowledge about Islam and access to the Islamic religious literature in the first decades of the twentieth century. They were skillful in drawing African Americans toward the mainstream Sunni Islam and to distance them from the nationalistic and anti-White connotations that were assumed in their early Muslim identity. Imam Warith Deen Muhammad (1933–2008) played a pivotal role in crystallizing and consolidating this paradigm shift in the African American Muslim community. Louis Farrakhan of the Nation of Islam is a representative of the latter, anti-White, form of Islam still practiced by a minority of African American Muslims.

A strong incentive for Muslim immigration to the United States was provided by the McCarran–Walter Act of 1952 that relaxed the quota system established in 1924, and a greater impetus was provided with the liberalization of the American immigration law in 1965. These revisions allowed Muslim immigrants opportunities to flee from oppressive regimes in many parts of the Muslim world, such as Syria, Lebanon, Albania, Yugoslavia, Egypt, Iran, and Palestine, who migrated in anticipation of better economic and educational opportunities, greater religious freedom, and family reunions. More recently, due to political upheavals, civil wars, and international wars, many new Muslim arrivals are from Somalia, Sudan, Afghanistan, former Yugoslavia, and the Persian Gulf. Based on surveys conducted by the Council on American-Islamic Relations, there were 962 mosques across the United States in 1994 and 1,209 in 2000 (CAIR 2001: 3). In 2007, the number rose to 1,250. In addition, there were approximately 2,000 Islamic centers and schools (CAIR 2007: 9). Islam is perhaps the third largest religion in America with major concentrations of Muslim population in the suburbs of major cities of the Northeast and Midwest, such as New York, Chicago, Detroit, and Dearborn, Michigan, and in other urban areas such as Houston, Los Angeles, San Francisco, and Cedar Rapids, Iowa. Muslims are also found in high concentration in states that have warm weather, such as Florida, Texas, Arizona, and California (Carroll 2000: 103).

In the early phase of its development, the Muslim community directed its energies into acquiring facilities to enable them to perform the devotional prayer services and commemorate significant religious events, such as the month of fasting and the festival of celebrating the conclusion of the month of fasting. Subsequently, they expanded their efforts to provide for religious training to the children, youth, and young adults and to ensure a proper knowledge base of Islam for all. In the 1980s, full-time accredited schools were established that provided one-hour daily instruction on the Qur'an, Islamic ethics, and the Islamic worldview. Subsequently, other agencies were established to provide services in marital counseling, parenting, and other religious issues.

In the post 9/11 context, Muslims and Arabs saw erosion of their civil rights and became targets of negative stereotypes and objects of ridicule and discrimination that became ingrained as a result of the negative portrayal of Islam and its demonization in the popular culture – music, cinema, television, and the print media. To deal with some of these issues, Muslims have begun to establish national, regional, and local Muslim institutions with the aim of providing a united voice on issues of shared concern – examples of such institutions are Muslim Public Affairs Council, Council on American-Islamic Relations, Muslim Students Association, Islamic Society of North America, Institute on Religion and Civil Values, and Council of Religious Scholars. Recently, Muslims have become active participants and promoters of interfaith dialogue that is governed by the principles of mutual respect and mutual enrichment. This constitutes a significant paradigm shift. Exclusivist claims of salvation have been toned down and greater efforts have been made in articulating points of convergence and commonalities among the various faith traditions. While Muslims have made substantial progress on the interfaith front, the critical importance of intra-Muslim discourse has only recently come to prominence with the upsurge in sectarian violence in Iraq that is framed as a Sunni–Shi'a, intra-Muslim feud. Another area where the egalitarian worldview of Islam is lacking is in the relationship between the immigrant Muslims and the indigenous African American Muslims, and in the area of gender equality. There is no denying that an element of racism is present in the Muslim community and this finds expression in the lack of inter-racial marriages and in the establishment of segregated ethnic-based Islamic centers in spite of the pluralistic nature of the American landscape. However, post 9/11, substantial efforts are being made to bridge the gap between the African American Muslims and the immigrant Muslims.

One of the major challenges and concerns that are faced by the Muslim community in America is alienation and disillusionment of its youth population from its religious and cultural roots. There is a disconnect between the imported religious leaders, who have been educated and trained abroad in the seminaries, and the Muslim youth population's concerns and issues. The transplanted religious leader may find the American society alien and lack the English language proficiency to be able to communicate effectively with the young population. In addition, many of these religious leaders are asked to perform tasks for which they have not been trained, such as the role of counselors, community activists, interfaith dialogue participants, fundraisers, and spokespersons for their respective communities and for the Muslims. Surprisingly, the 2007 Pew survey documented that younger Muslim Americans are more religiously observant and they are regular frequenters to the mosque in comparison to the older Muslims. In addition, a larger percentage of the younger Muslim Americans, especially among the African Americans, are displeased and disillusioned with the American system and are pessimistic of the future. This may be the outcome of the

9/11 catastrophic event and the subsequent circulation of the negative stereotypes of Muslims which has propelled young Muslims to assert their religious identity instead of their social identity.

The same Pew survey indicated that overall Muslims have a positive evaluation of the American public and society and view this land as one of actualizing one's potential with equity and fairness. Although many have been targets of discrimination and suspicion after 9/11 and vehemently oppose the war in Iraq, practically all (99 percent) are of the view that random acts of terrorism against innocent civilians are not justifiable.

Beliefs and practices

General

Embedded in the very word that describes the believer in Islam, "Muslim," is perhaps the single most important belief in the religion. Muslim means one who submits to God. Indeed, given the belief that all humans are a creation of God, in the worldview of Islam all humans are "muslim" at birth. Upon maturity and realization of one's dependence upon God, one then submits to his divinity and becomes Muslim. Typically, a verbal recognition of this submission is given in the statement "There is no god except God and Muhammad is the messenger of God." Essential to this recognition of God is a rejection of the idea that God is many; strict monotheism defines Islam.

Belief in Muhammad and his role as a messenger of God is also essential to Islam. He is seen as a prophet of the sort found in the pages of previous monotheistic revelations such as the Hebrew Bible. Thus he is seen in the line of the great prophets who brought forth significant religions and/or reform of religions, such as Noah, Abraham, Moses, and Jesus. All of these former prophets are to be honored, believed, and their messages respected, as Muhammad himself modeled. But Muhammad and God's revelation through him was specifically aimed at the people of Arabic descent present on what we now call the Saudi Arabian peninsula. The people there were thought to be ignorant of God and Muhammad's message brought them forth out of the ignorance that was marked by the worship of many idols whom they thought to be gods.

In addition to the effort to bring the people out of their polytheistic beliefs, Muhammad's message also urged them to accept the trust that God had given them as stewards of his creation. God desired that they serve as examples of how best to live justly and uphold God's desires for this world. Social justice was essential to Muhammad's early message as he and his followers put an end to the Arabic tribal practice of female infanticide and ownership of humans. In addition, while the Islamic faith expanded rapidly, there was to be no coercion exerted toward persons of other faiths. Should a person choose to submit to God this was celebrated. But all people who valued and practiced other religions were free to do so in Islamic society.

Authority in the growing Islamic faith settled upon two primary sources; the Qur'an and the life of Muhammad. His personal life, his practices, his character traits, and his teachings became exemplary for all Muslims. Over time, in addition to the Qur'an, the sayings of the Prophet became authoritative as well. Codified into volumes and traced back from witness to witness to the mouth of Muhammad, his words took on significant influence in the thinking of the religious leaders of Islam.

The daily lives of those who submit to God have also taken on particular patterns as the religion developed. These orthodox practices have come to be known as the Five Pillars of Islam. The first is that which was noted above, namely, the *shahada* or verbal testimony of one's belief in God and the Prophet. The second is the practice of daily prayers or *salat*; typically performed five times per day while facing Mecca. The third pillar is the giving of alms for the less fortunate, called in Arabic *zakat*. Fourth, and these are not intended in any sort of strict order of importance or priority, is the fast undertaken during the time of Ramadan. This is called *sawm* in Arabic. Fifth is the obligation to undertake the *Hajj* or religious pilgrimage in Saudi Arabia. Of course, if one is physically unable to manage the rigor of such a pilgrimage, or even that of Ramadan or the prostration of prayer, accommodation is immediate and widely understood.

These general beliefs provide the foundation and background for the faith community of Islam. Built upon these founding notions the leaders and faithful of Islam have established a large body of practices, both formal and informal, religious and cultural, upon which the faithful can rely for day-to-day living.

Health and disease

Islam's attitude toward sexual morality differs significantly from that of other religions and this is reflected in its stand on procreation, use of reproductive technologies, birth control, and abortion. The Qur'an and the prophetic literature provide a very positive evaluation of marriage as an institution that has been divinely blessed and highly encouraged. The primordial disposition for mutual attraction between the two sexes is natural and must be cultivated in such a way that it leads to a healthy marriage that will be permeated with love and mercy: "One of His signs is that He created spouses from among yourselves for you to live with in tranquility: He ordained love and kindness between you. In this truly are signs for those who reflect" (Qur'an 30:21). Detaching oneself away from the society as well as celibacy are denounced and viewed as reprehensible practices that should be avoided under normal circumstances. Prophet Muhammad is reported to have said: "Marriage is my tradition; whosoever dissociates from my tradition does not belong to me" (*Awali al-la'ali* 1983: 2:261). In another instance, he says: "Marry among yourselves and multiply, for I shall make a display of you before other nations on the Day of Judgment" (*Kanz al-'ummal* n.d.: 16:276). One of the primary reasons for marriage is procreation but it is not the sole reason because sexual gratification and companionship are also included without a negative connotation attached to them. However, infertility on the part of the woman is viewed as a deficiency and lowers her stature in the society. Accordingly, use of reproductive technologies to cure infertility would be welcomed, provided that it does not violate the other legal/moral/ethical rulings of Islam, such as using the sperm and/or the egg from a donor other than the married couple, surrogacy, viewing of the private organs by the opposite gender, use of frozen embryos where one or both of the previously married couple are dead or have become divorced, and so on (Mavani 1996: 51–2).

A gamut of opinions have been issued by Sunni jurists on surrogate maternity in a scenario of a polygamous relationship where one of the wives of the husband does not have a uterus to bring the pregnancy to term. A question was posed on whether embryo transfer between the wives of the same husband would be permissible and the responses range from permissible to absolutely prohibited. Likewise, diverse opinions are offered by Shi'i jurists. For instance, Ayatullah Sayyid Ali Sistani of Najaf, Iraq, permits the use of surrogate maternity provided that the artificial fertilization comprises the ovum and the sperm from the couple who are in a lawful marriage contract – be it permanent or temporary (Shi'i law permits very specific types of temporary, contractual marriage). Both the mother that provided the ovum and the surrogate mother would have claim over the child and thus he suggests, based on obligatory precaution, neither one of them should be excluded from this claim. Ayatullah Khamene'i of Iran goes even further by allowing for the donation of embryos of married couples to others who are legally married but unable to have children due to infertility provided that the latter obtain permission from the family court (Atighetchi 2007: 150).

The contraceptive practice of coitus interruptus (*'azl*) was used during the time of Prophet Muhammad and he never interjected to prohibit this practice. On the contrary, there is sufficient evidence to argue that he viewed the process of procreation exclusively in the hands of the Omnipotent God such that no human intervention can prevent the birth of a child if it has been divinely decreed. Jurists have extrapolated from this case and allowed the use of contraceptive devices, provided that they are not harmful for the women. However, most regard it to be reprehensible where one does not have a valid justification, such as economic hardship or time constraints that would not allow proper parental attention given to the character building of the child. One exception to this view is Ibn Hazm (994–1064), who viewed coitus interruptus as a form of camouflaged infanticide. Although there is a consensus on the employment of temporary forms of contraception, such is not the case when it comes to permanent contraception that cannot be reversed or the probability of reversal is negligible, such as vasectomy and tubal ligation. The latter is prohibited under normal conditions where the couple are healthy and not carriers of serious hereditary diseases that can be transmitted to the fetus.

In Sunni Islam, the issue of abortion is very much tied to defining the moment that the soul enters the developing fetus in the mother's womb. The story of creation in the Qur'an is explicit that humans attain personhood upon the infusion of the divine breath into their bodies or ensoulment of the fetus and, as a result, the angels are commanded to bow down out of reverence and respect for the humans: "When I have shaped him and breathed My Spirit into him, kneel down before him" (Qur'an 38:72). The statements of the prophet provide conflicting data on the precise time that the soul enters the fetus. However, the most recurring one is that the ensoulment takes place on the 120th day, or between 40 and 45 days from the date of fertilization. In cases where the mother's life is not at risk by bringing the pregnancy to term, jurists have been divided on the legality of aborting a fetus that is less than 120 days old – ranging from permission and discouragement, with a valid cause for terminating the pregnancy such as economic hardship, to outright prohibition. There is a development of a general trend in all the schools of thought within Sunni Islam to categorically prohibit abortion after 40 days have lapsed from the date of fertilization except in serious exigencies, such as saving the life of the mother. Although one can find diversity of opinions on abortion prior to the ensoulment of the soul, such is not the case in the period of post-ensoulment. There is almost unanimity on the absolute prohibition of abortion after the ensoulment of the fetus, except in a case where continuation of the pregnancy would be fatal for the mother or cause her serious mental and/or physical harm.

Among the four Sunni schools of law, the Hanafi legal school is most tolerant of abortion done before the ensoulment of the fetus. It is viewed as reprehensible and abominable, but still allowed with or without a valid reason. The Maliki school's position is very similar to the Twelver Shi'is in prohibiting abortion at any stage of the pregnancy except if warranted to save the life of the mother. The Shafi'i jurists have allowed abortion within the first 40 days, although it is given the moral value of *makruh* or strongly discouraged and detestable. The Hanbali legal school's position has varied from prohibition after conception to permission to abort, although morally reprehensible, the zygote in the first 40 days. In Shi'a Islam, abortion is prohibited at any stage after fertilization except in a case of therapeutic abortion to save the life of the mother.

The Qur'an speaks of the seven stages of embryonic development:

> We created man from an essence of clay, then We placed him as a drop of fluid in a safe place, then We developed that drop into a clinging form, and We developed that form into a lump of flesh, and We

developed that lump into bones, and We clothed those bones with
flesh, and later we developed him into other forms – glory be to God,
the best of creators! Then you will die and then, on the Day of Resurrection, you will be raised again.

(Qur'an 23:12–16)

Regardless of the specific issue at hand, it is generally important to keep in
mind the importance of the relationship between the care provider(s) and
the patient(s) in Islamic thought. Both Sunni and Shi'a Islam encourage the
scenario of same-sex provider–patient relationship. Put negatively, they
discourage the routine pairing of opposite sex provider with patients. This
concern to protect the virtue of both the provider and the patient is suspended in situations of emergency, but must be attended to in the routine
care of patients. Similarly important along these lines, when the situation
demands opposite-sex provider–patient relationships, providers should be
sure never to attend to patients without others present, be it family and/or
additional care providers.

Death and dying

Beliefs

There has been much discussion from the early period of Muslim history on
the question of free will and predestination. This theological discussion was
not strictly academic in nature; rather, it was organically related to the issue
of political legitimacy of the Umayyads who ruled the Muslim world from
661 to 750 CE. Most of the leaders or caliphs from this dynasty were of low
stature in character and are credited with minimal devotion to the dictates of
Islam. As a result, the community was engaged in evaluating the legality of
their status and whether a rebellion against them would be in conformity
with the Qur'an and the prophetic paradigm. The Umayyads were proponents of the theory of divine determinism to appease the community by providing religious reasoning that the role of leadership had been bestowed on
them based on divine decree and that all their actions were decreed by God.
Any attempt to overthrow them would constitute an act of sin and a challenge to the omnipotence and the comprehensive authority of God. This discussion took place in a context where the dominant view was one of fatalism
with a pessimistic notion of time as an inexorable force that will bring everything to an abrupt end. Death and destruction, fortune and misfortune, are
not categories where the humans have any agency. This particular understanding of human actions and the role of time in bringing about death at a
pre-determined date is mocked by the Qur'an:

They say, "There is only our life in this world: we die, we live, nothing
but Time destroys us." They have no knowledge of this; they only

follow guesswork: their only argument, when Our clear revelations are recited to them, is to say, "Bring back our forefathers if what you say is true." [Prophet], say, "It is God who gives you life, then causes you to die, and then He gathers you all to the Day of Resurrection of which there is no doubt, though most people do not comprehend."

(Qur'an 45:24–6)

In the place of such pessimism, absence of human volition in determining one's future, and lack of human accountability, and an afterlife, the Qur'an introduces the concept that the earthly life is a testing ground and a bridge that can lead one to a life of eternal bliss and joy in the hereafter provided that one lives her life in accordance with the divine prescriptions. The status of the human being was elevated to that of the deputy (*khalifah*) of God (a term the Qur'an uses at 2:30) who is commissioned to actualize the divine purpose on earth such that humans can move toward the attainment of perfection and the establishment of a just social, moral, ethical, and spiritual order to achieve felicity and prosperity in this life and in the after-life. Accordingly, the end of the terrestrial life does not bring an end to human history. Rather, life on earth is the period of cultivation such that virtuous deeds could bear fruits in the afterlife. In one of the traditions, Prophet Muhammad is reported to have said: "This life is a farm to culti-vate for the hereafter" (*Awali al-la'ali* 1983: 1:27).

According to the Qur'an, humans are composed of two contradictory elements: divine spirit (Qur'an 32:7) and mud or clay (Qur'an 3:59 and 7:12). The divine breath and the primordial nature (*fitrah*) generate motivation toward that which is lofty and sublime. The second ingredient, mud, tends the humans toward lowliness and unbridled fulfillment of base desires. The knowledge of good and evil has been transmitted to the humans by way of "revealed books" in the form of prophets, scriptures, primordial nature (*fitrah*) (Qur'an 91:8–9), and the book of nature, which point toward the existence of God who is worthy of adoration, worship, and submission (Qur'an 10:6–7). The freedom of choice that is enjoyed by humans elevates their status in relation to the angels. Accordingly, nobility is contingent upon the bestowal of free will and knowledge, and not on natural and racial characteristics. Humans are summoned by God to develop a bond with Him and perform noble deeds such that they can reap the rewards of their works in the afterlife.

Unlike in Christianity, there is no notion of original sin in Islam. On the contrary, one can make a case that there is a concept of original purity because every human being is born with an unadulterated conscience and a primordial disposition to abide by the universal moral and ethical values. In a prophetic tradition, Muhammad says: "Every child is born on his natural state of good conscience" (*al-Sunan al-kubra* n.d.: 6:203). The Qur'an is cognizant that humans have been created with inclination toward virtue but they are capable of going against this natural tendency and inevitably will fall prey to satanic temptations and, as a result, commit sins. However, all sins can be forgiven prior to the onset of death and loss of agency (Qur'an 39:53 and 4:31), including the greatest sin of polytheism or associationism (*shirk*) (Qur'an 4:48), provided the person sincerely seeks forgiveness, renounces the evil act, regenerates virtuous desires and intentions, and provides restitution to the wronged party. The first moral/ethical violation of Adam and Eve, the first humans as told in the Qur'an, took the form of eating from the forbidden tree at the prompting of Satan (Qur'an 7:20–2 and 20:121). Thereafter, both of them sought God's forgiveness for this error of judgment and were forgiven: "Then Adam received some words from his Lord and He accepted his repentance: He is the Ever Relenting, the Most Merciful" (Qur'an 2:37). Thus, there is no transmission of "original error" or "sin" to their posterity, or a permanent abandonment from God.

As mentioned above, in the Islamic tradition, life on earth is viewed as a prelude and a precursor to the eternal life in the hereafter, and a preparatory phase before returning back to our origin: "We belong to God and to Him we shall return" (Qur'an 2:157). The inevitability of death and the ultimate return to God for accountability and meeting Him is underlined in the Qur'an in various places. The major phases of a human being from non-existence to resurrection are discussed as follows: "How can you ignore God when you were lifeless and He gave you life, when He will cause you to die, then resurrect you to be returned to Him?" (Qur'an 2:28).

God is the one who inspired his divine breath into human beings and gave him life, dignity, and trusteeship over their bodies. This trust is not absolute, just as human ownership of worldly things is not absolute. Accordingly, issues that deal with the termination of life require the consent and the endorsement of the absolute Trustee and Creator of human life.

The matter of defining the exact point when life commences and terminates is fraught with difficulties and challenges because the revelatory sources are not explicit in its articulation. However, one thing is clear, that God is the author of life and death. It is possible to find verses in the Qur'an that speak of a pre-determined term of life or on the date of death just as humankind's sustenance has already been pre-recorded: "No person grows old or has his life cut short, except in accordance with a Record: all this is easy for God" (Qur'an 35:11) and "No soul may die except with God's permission at a predestined time" (Qur'an 3:145). Works that deal with death have as their focus the soul after having separated from the body. Not much attention is paid to defining the moment of death other than in general terms, such as the parting of the soul from the body. However, in Islamic legal theory there is a basic rule that the jurists should defer to experts in the field concerned for authoritative understanding of the definition within that particular field. So, for instance, the jurist would rely on experts to identify the direction for the shortest distance to Mecca in order to offer the daily ritual prayers and for positioning the deceased in the grave. Likewise, it would be customary to rely upon astronomical evidence to ascertain the birth of a new crescent when the conditions are such that the moon is blocked by clouds. Accordingly, in determining the valid criteria of death, jurists need to seek counsel and advice of doctors. Traditional signs of discerning death by external evidences were largely derived from human experience and are not of great relevance in light of the ability of modern technology to sustain some form of organ activity.

Upon the onset of death, it is recommended to perform certain rituals in order to facilitate ease of departure of the soul from the patient's body, to safeguard it from undergoing hardship and torment, and to re-confirm the covenant of the patient with the Creator by reciting the dual testimony of faith: there is no god except one God and Muhammad is the messenger of God. During this time, rules of segregation and modesty must be adhered to between the male and the female. Family members must be informed of the impending death of the patient so that they can be close for comfort and solace. They also encourage the patient to seek repentance from God for lapses and petition God to forgive. It is discouraged and reprehensible to leave the dying patient alone or to weep and wail uncontrollably because this would imply a lack of resignation to God's decree for the appointed time of death. In addition, it is customary to recite certain chapters of the Qur'an, such as Yasin (verse 36) and the Confederates (verse 33), and to remind the dying of the covenant with God and his messenger and, in Shi'ism, also with the 12 infallible imams or guides. It is recommended to position the dying person such that her soles would be facing the Ka'bah in Mecca, which is the same direction that Muslims offer their five daily ritual prayers. The patient, once deceased, can be left in that state until taken away for the ritual washing, funeral prayers, and burial. In Sunni Islam, it is also accepted that the body can be laid at a perpendicular angle such that the Ka'bah is to the right of the dying person. In the Muslim tradition, it is believed that one who has lived a life anchored in moral and ethical worldview and has rendered beneficial services to humanity will be greeted by the angel of death with the following words: "O you, soul at peace: return to your Lord well pleased and well pleasing; Go in among My servants, and into My Garden" (Qur'an 89:27–30).

Upon the death of the patient, one should close the mouth, fasten the two jaws with a strip of cloth so that the mouth will not open up, straighten the hands and the legs, cover the corpse with a clean sheet of cloth, and pray. The dead body must be treated with respect and dignity because it is argued that it can still feel the pain as the soul still has affinity to it. The rules of modesty of the deceased Muslim woman must be adhered to as if she were alive. It is critically important to avoid delaying the ritual of washing, shrouding, praying, and burying the deceased. Consequently, arrangements ought to be made to expeditiously fulfill the necessary religious requirements, and this would normally be carried out by the person who has been delegated by the deceased. Responsibility of providing the burial services to the deceased devolves upon all the Muslims, but as soon as someone or a group has fulfilled this obligation, others would be exempted. However, if none were to provide the burial services, then all would be guilty of having committed a sin and religiously accountable for this moral violation. If the deceased is a child of four months or less, there is no ritual washing, shrouding, and offering of ritual prayers. Instead, the child is wrapped up in a piece of cloth and then buried.

After the deceased has been washed, shrouded, prayed over, and buried, Islamic tradition states that, on the first night after the burial, the soul will re-enter the body so that he/she can be questioned by two angels – *Munkar* and *Nakir* – on their testimony of faith in God and His messenger (and in Shi'ism the 12 divine guides as well), the Scripture, the angels, and the Day of Accountability. If successful, the grave will be expanded and made spacious, and the deceased will be able to smell the breeze from paradise until the day of resurrection. If unsuccessful, the grave will become narrow and torment, as a foretaste of the punishment in the hell-fire, will commence. This period is known as *barzakh*, the barrier between death and resurrection or the intermediate world of imagination.

Practices

The Qur'an is explicit and unambiguous in its assertion that the originator of life is God and only God has the prerogative to terminate it. As a matter of fact, the term of each individual has already been pre-determined and recorded: "[Prophet], say, 'It is God who gives you life, then causes you to die, and then He gathers you all to the Day of Resurrection of which there is no doubt, though most people do not comprehend'" (Qur'an 45:26). The misguided idea that one can delay the appointed time of death is denounced as a show of human arrogance: "Death will overtake you no matter where you may be, even inside high towers" (Qu'ran 4:78). This is not intended to generate a feeling of fatalism; rather, it is a reflection of the all-comprehensive authority and knowledge of God who is aware of all that is to transpire on the basis of human free will.

The prohibition of suicide in Islam is based on the notion that life is sacred and that it is a divine trust that God has bestowed on human beings. Violation of this trust and arrogation of God's position as the author of life and death would constitute arrogance and an expression of ingratitude to God's favors and bounties. The commission of suicide in the face of despondency and hopelessness would be equally condemned because this would be a reflection of ungratefulness and inability to resign to the divine will. As a result, suicide falls under the category of major sins. The Prophet is reported to have said that one who is guilty of suicide will be subject to eternal punishment by being consigned to the hell-fire forever without any chance of a reprieve. The Scripture admonishes the humans not to be the source of its own destruction: "Spend in God's cause: do not contribute to your destruction with your own hands, but do good, for God loves those who do good" (Qur'an 2:195).

Life on earth is viewed as a testing ground where humans will be afflicted with trials and tribulation in the form of loss of lives, property, and economic stability: "We shall certainly test you with fear and hunger, and loss of property, lives, and crops. But [Prophet], give good news to those who are steadfast" (Qur'an 2:155). Human suffering may not be explicable to the limited faculty of human reason. However, there always exists a rationale and wisdom because God is not capricious and unkind to mete out hardship without a purpose. Some prophetic traditions make references to cleansing of one's sins or providing an example for the living as possible reasons for undergoing the calamities. The ability to endure these challenges with patience and forbearance is a sign of strong conviction.

At the same time, employment of palliative care to reduce the suffering and improve the quality of life is encouraged. In early Islamic legal literature, active forms of euthanasia or physician-assisted suicide were often equated with suicide with little or no distinction made between the two, and the same holds true in contemporary times. Present-day scholars do implicitly allow for passive forms of euthanasia by interpreting this posture as a sign of one's resignation to the divine will which determines the final outcome. This position can be further buttressed by arguing that artificially delaying an inevitable death by recourse to invasive procedures is contrary to the interest of the patient to die with dignity when the life has no longer any merit, whether to self or to society. This ruling can be applied in the case of brain-dead patients or situations where there is no hope of survival so that they are allowed to die by recourse to a passive form of euthanasia whether by not providing certain treatments that would have only delayed the imminent death, by not connecting the patient to a life-saving apparatus, or by administering drugs that alleviate pain but may accelerate the patient's death. There is lack of unanimity among the Twelver Shi'i jurists on the legality of withdrawing the life-support apparatus once it has already been connected to the patient and activated. The breakneck pace of advances in medical technology will force the jurists to provide new definitions of death. It goes without saying that all decisions made by physicians require the consent of the patient and the immediate family or the person designated to make decisions on the patient's behalf.

In the Islamic tradition, the body is accorded respect, dignity, and honor even after the soul has departed from it. As such, in order to preserve the integrity of the body it was prohibited to subject it to an autopsy or post-mortem investigation, to donate organs, or to use body organs to advance science in finding cures for the many ailments. All these practices were viewed as disfiguring of a corpse and violating the dignity of the deceased. However, the principle of public welfare (*maslahah*) where the benefits outweigh the demerits has allowed for a re-evaluation of the Islamic ruling on these issues. Even then, the jurists were still mindful of the sanctity of the body of a believer and thus would counsel that their bodies be spared if there are volunteers among the unbelievers who would fulfill the need. However, an ethical problem arises when one attempts to sustain such a view, particularly in light of the notion of universal human dignity that is vouched in the Qur'anic verse: "We have honored the children of Adam and carried them by land and sea" (Qur'an 17:71). Thus, some jurists have further revised their opinions and argued that all life is equally precious and thus no distinctions ought to be made between the believers and the unbelievers. In the case of autopsy, it would be permitted if it is mandated by the law of the land or the merits outweigh the demerits. Cremation, on the other hand, is strictly prohibited and is not open for discussion or analysis.

Conclusion

Given the conjoined seminal history of the Abrahamic faiths, it should not be surprising that so much of what we have learned in this chapter on Islam is similar to what we find in Judaism and Christianity. Aside from the variety of positions we see within Islam, the general frame of reference to God and his revealed word through Prophet Muhammad remains central. Healthcare professionals who are respectful of the seriousness with which Muslims practice their faith will be a step ahead. Granting respect to the person who identifies with Islam, whether in past family or cultural connections or in present-day involvement, is essential in the effort to properly care for patients.

Table 9.1 Dos and don'ts

Dos	Don'ts
1 Ask if the patient would like privacy to pray.	1 Do not feed the patient anything that contains pork or any porcine by-products, such as lard.
2 Ask if the patient would prefer providers of a specific gender.	2 Do not assume religious traditions are not of concern.
3 Ask if the patient would like help contacting the local imam.	3 Do not assume that prayer is not a concern while in the hospital.
4 Make sure the dietician is aware of food consumption rules.	4 Do not send an opposite-sex caregiver into the patient's room alone.
5 Make sure family is included in decision-making discussions.	

Case study

SD was a 13-year-old Sunni Muslim girl with leukemia who had undergone a bone marrow transplant. Her parents were of Pakistani background though she had been born in the United States. Sadly, her leukemia had relapsed and she was undergoing further chemotherapy. Her prognosis was poor. Because of her immunosuppression, SD developed an overwhelming infection with gram negative bacteria causing septic shock and difficulties breathing. Her kidney function also began to deteriorate and she was becoming more fluid overloaded. She was transferred from the Hematology/Oncology ward to the Pediatric Intensive Care Unit (PICU). The PICU team knew her well as they had provided sedation for her many oncology related procedures. Shortly after transfer to the PICU she needed more oxygen and it became clear that she might need intubation and mechanical ventilation. The family did not want us to talk directly to her about her condition, preferring instead that we process all information through them. Some members of the PICU team voiced their concern with intubating her in light of her poor prognosis but the family wished to proceed. SD was intubated and placed on heavy sedation because of her constant struggling against the ventilator. A bone marrow biopsy performed a few days later offered no definitive answer about the continued presence of her leukemia. Her kidney function worsened and thus she needed dialysis. She required multiple blood transfusions for low blood counts and liver insufficiency. She began to uncontrollably bleed from her mouth and nose. The PICU team believed dialysis could be withheld as her prognosis was so poor with her ongoing multi-organ failure. The family did not agree to this limitation as they believed there was still a possibility that the cancer could be gone. They said, "Allah will let us know when it is her time". They had discussed her condition with many family members and local imams, including the imam of the mosque in the father's hometown in Pakistan. The community opinion was that only Allah decides when it is time for death. A hemodialysis catheter was placed and continuous dialysis was begun. Local Muslims began visiting frequently, saying prayers at the bedside and reciting Qu'ran. The father's brother came from Pakistan to offer support. Over the next few weeks, SD's condition worsened and she became more swollen and discolored. An additional bone marrow biopsy remained inconclusive due to acellularity. Do Not Attempt Resuscitation (DNAR) code status was discussed with the family but the mother refused as she clung to the possibility that if the cancer was no longer present every effort should be made to keep her alive. The family requested the opinion of a Muslim doctor in the hospital, who shared her concern about the overall prognosis of the child and prolongation of suffering. The doctor pointed out that in the face of medical futility it was permissible in Islam to limit therapies. Again, the PICU team expressed discomfort in prolonging SD's situation. Approximately a month following her admission to the

PICU, SD developed septic shock once more. Her heart function began to worsen and inotropic support was increased. As her cell count was now elevated, another bone marrow biopsy was completed and the results showed the presence of cancer cells. The family asked to speak to the Muslim doctor once more; since the leukemia was back the parents agreed to DNAR and discontinuation of dialysis. They believed Allah had guided them to this decision. SD died a few days later with comfort measures in place and the family at her bedside.

Questions for reflection

1   Must ICU care teams always do what families request of them? Could there be situations when the care team simply refuses to do what the family asks?
2   Should requests for faith-specific physicians (or any caregiver) be honored by hospitals?
3   Putting yourself in the position of the Muslim MD, knowing your tradition allows for discontinuation of life-sustaining measures in the face of medical futility, how would you counsel the parents? What, exactly, would you say in response to the faith statement that Allah/God decides when people die?

Glossary

Hadith   The sayings of the Prophet Muhammad written down later by his closest associates and catalogued by the faith community.

Hajj   The pilgrimage that each Muslim believer is encouraged to undertake at least once in her/his life, if able. Presently, yearly, over one million faithful make the pilgrimage from Medina to Mecca in Saudi Arabia.

Haram   An action that is forbidden under a fivefold designation of all human actions in Islamic thought. The other four are: *wajib* (obligatory), *mandub* (recommended), *mubah* (permissible or neutral), and *makruh* (reprehensible or discouraged).

Imam   The title of respect used for the leader of the local community of Muslim believers. Parallel terms in Judaism and Christianity, respectively, would be: rabbi and pastor or priest.

Ka'bah   The place of worship originally constructed by Abraham and his son Ishmael. It is the place toward which all faithful Muslims face when they pray. At the end of the Hajj, the pilgrims circumambulate the Ka'bah together.

Qur'an   Holy scripture in the Islamic religion. It was given to Muhammad with the idea of ending the time of ignorance for the Arabic tribes of his day.

Ramadan   An annual time of religious and personal devotion during the ninth month of the Muslim calendar. Muslims who are able must fast from all food and water during the day time. Fast is broken after the sunset and families enjoy delightful meal times together.

Sunnah   The Sunnah is the record of the words and deeds of Prophet Muhammad, including for Shi'a Muslims the words and deeds of his designated successors. Along with the Qur'an, the Sunnah constitutes the second major source of authority for Islamic law.

Bibliography

Ahmad b. al-Husayn b. 'Ali al-Bayhaqi (n.d.) *al-Sunan al-kubra*, 10 vols, Beirut: Dar al-fikr.

al-Mar'ashi, al-S. and al-Araqi, al-S. M. (eds) (1983) Ibn Abi Jumhur al-Ahsa'i, *Awali al-la'ali*, 4 vols, Qum: Sayyid al-shuhada'.

al-Muttaqi al-Hindi (n.d.) *Kanz al-'ummal*, 16 vols, Beirut: Mu'assasat al-risalah.

Atighetchi, D. (2007) *Islamic Bioethics: Problems and Perspectives*, New York: Springer.

Carroll, B. (2000) "Islam in America," in *The Routledge Historical Atlas of Religion in America*, New York: Routledge, p. 103.

Counsel on American-Islamic Relations (CAIR) (2001) *The Mosque in America: A National Portrait*, Washington, DC: CAIR. Available online at: www.cair.com/images/pdf/The-American-mosque-2001.pdf (accessed October 4, 2016).

Counsel on American-Islamic Relations (CAIR) (2007) *Sharing Ramadan: Resource Guide 2007*, Washington, DC: CAIR. Available online at: www.cair.com/pdf/SharingRamadanResourceGuide2007.pdf (accessed December 11, 2008).

Leonard, K. I. (2003) *Muslims in the United States: The State of Research*, New York: Russell Sage Foundation, p. 4.

Mavani, H. (tr.) (1996) Ayatullah Sayyid Ali Sistani, *Contemporary Legal Rulings in Shi'i Law*, Montreal: OAIK Publications, pp. 51–2, questions 137a and b.

Nekola, A. (2011). *Muslim Americans: No Signs of Growth in Alienation or Support for Extremism*, Pew Research Center. Available online at: www.people-press.org/2011/08/30/muslim-americans-no-signs-of-growth-in-alienation-or-support-for-extremism/ (accessed May 31, 2016).

Pew Research Center (2007) *Muslim Americans: Middle Class and Mostly Mainstream*. Available online at: http://pewresearch.org/pubs/483/muslim-americans (accessed December 11, 2008).

Suggested texts

Abdel Haleem. M. A. S. (tr.) (2004) *The Qur'an: A New Translation*, Oxford: Oxford University Press.

Ahmed, L. (1993) *Women and Gender in Islam: Historical Roots of a Modern Debate*, New Haven: Yale University Press.

Hodgson, M. G. S. (1977) *The Venture of Islam*, 3 vols, Chicago: University of Chicago Press.

Lings, M. (2006) *Muhammad: His Life Based on the Earliest Sources*, rev. edn, Rochester, VT: Inner Traditions.

Rahman, F. (1998) *Health and Medicine in the Islamic Tradition: Change and Identity*, Chicago: Kazi Publications.

Sachedina, A. (2009) *Islamic Biomedical Ethics: Principles and Application*, Oxford: Oxford University Press.

10 Judaism

Douglas Kohn

Hear O Israel, Adonai is our God, Adonai is one.

Deuteronomy 6:4

I call heaven and earth to witness before you this day, that I have set before you life and death, the blessing and the curse; therefore choose life that you may live.

Deuteronomy 30:19

Introduction

Judaism, the oldest monotheistic religious system and the first textually-based religion in the Western world, has a fundamental identification and concern with life, health, and healing. At the crowning climax of the Hebrew Bible's opening chapter (Genesis 1:26–28), God formed humankind (*Adam*) in the Divine Image and charged the nascent humanity to procreate and to bear stewardship over the newly created earth. Thereafter, in the succeeding chapter which elucidates the initial creation mythology, one reads that God "breathed life into the man's nostrils" (Genesis 2:7), reflecting the Deity's intimacy with humanity and fundamental ethic of concern for the life and well-being of the human being, and by extension, the human enterprise. Yet, human life, by definition, is fragile and vulnerable, and invariably the living being requires care, mediation, and support. The text of Leviticus 19:16, "Do not stand idly by the blood of your neighbor," is interpreted to compel tending and healing of the ill or injured person.

Later, in the rabbinic teachings of the Talmud (the fifth century CE code of Jewish law), the creation of Adam again is invoked to promote the primary Jewish principle of the value of life:

> Therefore only a single human being was created in the world, to teach that if any person causes a single soul to perish, Scripture regards him as if he has destroyed an entire world; and if any person saves a single soul, Scripture regards him as if he had saved an entire world.
>
> (Babylonian Talmud [BT] *Sanhedrin* 37a)

This central concept of reverence for life finds further emphasis in the liturgy for the Jewish High Holy Days of *Rosh Hashanah* (the Jewish New Year) and *Yom Kippur* (the Day of Atonement), which reads, "In the book of life ... may we and all Your people ... be inscribed for a good and peaceful life" (Greenberg and Levine 1978: 181). One reads in the Midrash to the Hebrew Bible (a homiletic explication of the biblical text) the model of God visiting and comforting Abraham when the patriarch was healing from his circumcision (Genesis 17:26–18:1, BT *Sotah* 14a), demonstrating that the process of healing is a relational, cooperative endeavor, including possibly the presence of the Holy One, but surely, human contact. Lastly, in the final book of the Torah (also known as the Pentateuch or the Five Books of Moses) is found perhaps the most commanding verse authorizing a medical ethic and the religious charge to pursue healing and life: "I call heaven and earth to witness before you this day, that I have set before you life and death, the blessing and the curse; therefore choose life that you may live" (Deuteronomy 30:19). These textual references represent but a fraction of Jewish sacred scripture which serves as the foundation for a Jewish ethos of health and healing, yet each captures the common thrust: that life is cherished, and that the *mitzvah* (Divinely commanded obligation) to heal is a principle cornerstone of Jewish behavior and understanding.

One might note the large number of Jews engaged in the healing professions – as physicians, researchers, instructors, and therapists – both presently and historically, to realize the powerful influence which this ethic holds on the Jewish community. Furthermore, the Talmud teaches that it is forbidden to live in a community which lacks a physician, further compelling Jews to engage in the healing arts (BT *Sanhedrin* 17a). As much as Judaism commands the obligation to heal, it concomitantly commands the Jew to seek healing (Bleich 1981: 1–9).

Yet, Jews and Judaism are not monolithic. There is a great variety and breadth to the Jewish world and its community, with sub-streams of Jewry today spanning from the Orthodox and ultra-Orthodox sects at one extreme to Progressive and even secular Jewish streams at the opposite pole. Primarily, adherents within these Jewish sub-groups are distinguished in their respective practice and relationship to *halacha* (Jewish law), and less so in core ethics or beliefs. Some of these differences will be evident in postures toward health and medical circumstances. For the purposes of this chapter, a normative understanding and common practice are described, while noting important variations or minority examples.

Demographics

In 2010, the North American Jewish Data Bank estimated that the worldwide Jewish population numbered approximately 13.4 million persons, although there are estimates which suggest the Jewish population could number 14 or 15 million, due to some uncertainty in measurements and definitions. Of this population, approximately 43 percent, or nearly six million Jews, live in the State of Israel, and another 40 percent live in the United States. It is estimated that there are about 205,000 Jews in Russia, 483,500 in France, 375,000 in Canada, and 292,000 in the United Kingdom.

The same institute's study indicates that metropolitan areas with significant Jewish communities include Tel Aviv (three million), New York City (two million), Haifa (671,400) Jerusalem (703,600), Los Angeles (684,950), Paris (284,000), Moscow (95,000), Philadelphia (263,800), and London (195,000) (Della Pergola 2010).

Worldwide, two major branches represent the Jewish community of faith, the Orthodox and the Progressive, with significant sub-divisions in each branch. In the United States, the Progressive Jewish community is primarily comprised of the Reform Movement and the Conservative Movement, with Jews of the Reconstructionist and Renewal movements representing a small fraction of Progressive Jews. The National Jewish Population Study of 2000–2001 revealed that 35 percent of America's Jews identify as Reform (2,000,000), 26 percent identify as Conservative (1,500,000), 10 percent as Orthodox (600,000), and the remainder as "just Jewish" (United Jewish Communities 2001). In Israel and Europe, there is only one progressive movement, commonly called "Progressive Judaism." In Israel, it is estimated that 10 percent of Jews are ultra-Orthodox, 10 percent are Progressive, and the remainder are "just Jewish," which includes a mix of Orthodox and secular Jews. In Europe, a similar ratio is found, with a smaller fraction each of Orthodox and Progressive, and the majority in the middle. Worldwide, Orthodoxy is not monolithic, either. At its extreme, small numbers of Jews are *Haredi* or *Chasidic* Jews, who adhere to a very strict, medieval interpretation of Jewish law, while the bulk are "Modern Orthodox," who fully function in modern society while maintaining Jewish ritual.

The fastest growing stream in the United States is the Reform Movement, which has been moving in its practice and philosophy nearer to the Conservative Movement, such that in many communities there is little difference between the two major movements. In America, Modern Orthodoxy is losing members, while the ultra-Orthodox is growing due to its much greater birthrate. These trends also hold in Israel, though its Progressive Movement is growing more slowly.

History

Jewish history dates to the biblical period, or the early second millennium BCE. The patriarch, Abraham (*c.*1750 BCE), is credited with being the first Jew, and from him Jewry initially grew as a familial clan of adherents to the One God, known by the Hebrew tetragrammaton (the four-letter name of God in Hebrew language), YHWH, pronounced *"Adonai"* in Hebrew, the religious language of Judaism. An initial covenant was established, linking for perpetuity this people, God, and the land of Israel. Jewish patriarchal history is detailed in the biblical book of Genesis. After a period of Egyptian enslavement, the Jews were liberated by God through the hand of Moses, known as the lawgiver (*c.*1225 BCE), and they began a journey to return to their homeland. Essential to the journey was the revelation and renewed covenant at Sinai, at which Jewish tradition credits God with giving the Torah, containing 613 commandments.

Later biblical history includes the conquest of Canaan by Joshua, Moses' successor, and the period of kings who secured and enlarged the Jewish territory, later called Judea and Samaria. King David (*c.*1000 BCE) is the most celebrated of Israel's rulers. Concurrent with the period of the monarchies was the period of the prophets, the ethical teachers who tempered the rule of the kings and spoke as intermediaries for God. Isaiah, Jeremiah, Micah, and Ezekiel are the most heralded prophets. In the sixth century BCE, the Babylonians invaded Judea and destroyed the great temple in Jerusalem, the physical and emotional center of the Jewish faith. The Babylonians returned to their homeland with the Jews in tow as prisoners. The Jewish people refer to this as the Exile, which continued until the Jews returned later that century and built the Second Temple. Jewry endured Persian and then Greek rule until the end of the second century BCE, and then revolted against the Hellenized Assyrians in the uprising which would produce the festival of Chanukah.

The Rabbinic Period commenced with the Roman Period (*c.*63 BCE–500 CE), and the Roman destruction of the Second Temple. Central to the Rabbinic Period was the discourse of the rabbis, who generated a portable, textually-based religion which superseded the site-based ritualistic traditions of the Temples. The rabbis canonized the Bible, prepared the Jewish prayer book, set the festival and life cycle sequences, and wrote two codes of Jewish law, the Mishnah (redacted *c.*200 CE) and the Talmud (redacted *c.*500 CE). Essentially, the rabbis created Judaism as it is understood today. Also with the rabbinic period came the Diaspora, or the dispersion, as Jews spread to every corner of the Roman Empire, then to all over the globe until the modern period.

For the next 1,000 years, Jews remained a minority culture under the Muslim hegemony in the Mediterranean region and the Near East, and in Christian Europe from Iberia and North Africa to Persia and India, and throughout Europe. Jews learned to live under both cultural norms. As a literate minority in the societies where they lived, Jews often served as bureaucrats, diplomats, accountants, lawyers, and physicians in both Christendom and the Muslim worlds, although Jewry was relegated to secondary status in both societies. For Jews, the height of this period was the Golden Age of Spain (*c.*900–1200 CE), during which Jews were found in the royal courts, and were the doctors and poets of the Spanish kingdoms. In 1492, King

Ferdinand and Queen Isabella expelled the Jews from Spain, ending one of the greatest periods of Jewish history. The Jews of Spain, called Sephardic Jews, then emigrated and joined Jewish communities in the Mediterranean basin, and central and Eastern Europe (this later group being referred to as Ashkenazic, or German Jews).

With the modern world, Jews eventually were "liberated" and granted citizenship in the newly-formed nation-states of Europe and America. In the nineteenth century, the largest population of Jews was the Ashkenazim of Eastern Europe, living in Poland and Russia's Pale of Settlement (a region in Russia where Jews settled and later were persecuted). As well, there were sizable communities in Germany and Western Europe. Due to periodic pogroms (state-sanctioned violence against Jews in the nineteenth and early twentieth centuries), many Jews immigrated to America. The tragedy of the Holocaust (1938–1945, *Sho'a*, in Hebrew), during which the Nazis murdered six million Jews, resulted in nearly every European Jewish community being decimated and nearly every Jewish family suffering losses. Following the liberation of the death camps in Europe, American Jewry would be the world's largest Jewish community. In 1948, the State of Israel was established, and Israel absorbed over a million Jewish refugees from both Europe and the Arab states. Israel would share hegemony with American Jewry and would begin to generate its own, unique Jewish customs and traditions, including reviving Hebrew as a primary spoken tongue – 2,000 years after it was previously used as the language of Jews during the biblical and Rabbinic periods.

Beliefs and practices

General

Judaism is a system of deed, not creed. Although Judaism does include a number of central tenets, its fundamental system is one of commanded actions, not commanded beliefs. Of the 613 commandments given in the Hebrew Bible, all are charges of behavior, not of faith or precept. Hence, Judaism is not a faith-system, as most Western religions are termed, but a system of commandments, or *mitzvot*. The *mitzvot* may be categorized as either ritual commandments or as ethical commandments. Examples of ritual commandments include observance of Shabbat (the Sabbath), animal sacrifice for expiation of sins and guilt, dietary laws, and the obligation to circumcise eight-day-old boys. Examples of ethical commandments include honoring father and mother, leaving the corners of one's field for the hungry, not taking bribes, and respecting one's employees.

Despite this primary emphasis on behavior, beliefs are important. Judaism's fundamental belief is that God is one. Considered the central statement of Judaism, called the *shema* (meaning: "Hear"), Deuteronomy 6:4 states, "Hear O Israel, Adonai is our God, Adonai is one." Judaism, therefore, is the first monotheistic religion and makes the singularity and uniqueness of God its chief theme. Rejection of any suggestion of multiple gods, or of the divisibility of God, is central to Judaism and distinguishes Judaism from other religions. The idea of the oneness of God was further developed by the twelfth-century Jewish philosopher and physician in Spain, Moses Maimonides, also known as the Rambam. Arguably, he was the greatest Jewish theologian and the most celebrated medieval medical practitioner. In his commentary on the Mishnah, Maimonides posited 13 principles of faith, asserting the existence, unity, incorporeality, and eternity of God – that God alone is to be worshipped and that God knows human behavior and metes reward and punishment, including the resurrection of the dead. Today, most Jews still adhere to the Rambam's initial principles, but far fewer accept the latter concepts.

A second essential precept of Judaism is the covenantal relationship (*brit*) between God and the people of Israel. God established the covenant with Abraham recorded in chapters 12 and 17 of Genesis, which declared that God would be God to the people of Israel, would bless them with plentiful progeny, and would give them the land of Canaan. For their part, the people would keep the commandments for every generation. The covenant would be renewed at Mount Sinai (Exodus 19 and 20), and the symbol of the covenant would be the circumcision of the foreskin of all Jewish males.

Judaism professes values of the sanctity of life and respect for the body. Of all the commandments in the Torah, all except three of them (the prohibitions on murder, rape, and idolatry) may be violated for the sake of saving a life. This principle is called *piku'ah nefesh* (priority of saving a life). Existent life has priority over potential life. When necessary, a Jew may take risks for life, but is not required to risk his or her own life to save another. For instance, the Talmud discusses a situation when one may enter a burning building to save a life or the hypothetical case of travelers in the desert who must share a single flask of water. It teaches that one is not compelled to surrender oneself for the other. As well, because existent life has priority over potential life, when in conflict, the life of a pregnant mother takes precedence over that of the fetus. Judaism asserts the sanctity of the body, which is considered a sacred vessel of life and a gift from God. Thus, defacing the body, such as via tattoos or cutting, is prohibited as disrespect of God's gift. Likewise, Judaism also has disallowed autopsies or embalming, as each requires disfigurement of the body, and has formerly forbidden organ donation on the same grounds. Yet, after anti-rejection drugs, such as cyclosporine, have proven organ transplantation viable, rabbinic authorities have recanted their opposition on grounds of *piku'ah nefesh* – that for the sake of saving a life, the body of a deceased individual may be violated.

Judaism's festival sequence follows its particular, lunar calendar, with each day commencing and ending at sundown. Every seventh day at sunset, on Friday evening, commences *Shabbat* (the Sabbath), when Jews attend worship services at the synagogue and enjoy a festive *Shabbat* dinner. The Sabbath day, or Saturday, is a time of worship, study, rest, and family gathering. Key holy days include *Rosh Hashanah*, the Jewish New Year, and *Yom Kippur*, the Day of Atonement on which Jews fast to atone for misdeeds; these are the High Holy Days which occur in the early fall. The three biblical agricultural festivals of *Sukkot* (the fall harvest festival), Passover (*Pesach*, marking the exodus from Egypt), and *Shavuot* (commemorating the receipt of Torah at Sinai) are the major seasons of Jewish life and are treated as sacred days when the Jew abstains from work and worships in the synagogue. The eight-day winter celebration of Chanukah and the one-day spring festival of Purim mark Jewish victories over oppressors and include special foods. As well at Chanukah, Jews kindle an eight-branched candelabrum for eight nights. Besides *Yom Kippur*, there are other fast days in the Jewish calendar, most notably *Tisha B'Av*, which marks the destruction of the ancient temples. Out of mournfulness, Jews refrain from eating on such days. Also, Passover includes its own dietary restrictions, forbidding leavened foodstuffs and most grain products for the festival's eight days.

Kashrut (meaning "fit") is the name of the Jewish dietary system. Foodstuffs which are deemed proper for eating are called *kosher*, and those which are disallowed are termed *treif* (meaning "torn," i.e., the animal was killed by a predator and found in a field "torn"). Generally, animals whose meat is allowed are those mammals which chew their cud and have cloven, split hoofs. Hence, cattle and goats are allowed and are kosher, while pigs and dogs are disallowed. Permissible fish are those which have both fins and scales. Thus, catfish, which lack scales, and shellfish, which lack fins, are forbidden. Regarding fowl, the Torah lists those birds which are *kosher* and those which are *treif*, though basically predators and birds which eat carrion are *treif*. Also, in elucidating the Torah's laws of *kashrut*, the rabbis of the Talmud forbade mixing meat and milk in any individual meal. Thus, a cheeseburger or drinking milk with a chicken dish is *treif*. Some misinterpret the laws of *kashrut*, arguing that the rationale for these ancient precepts is concern for cleanliness and health. Although one may rightly argue that many of the forbidden animals may be unclean and may likely propagate disease, there is no evidence that such concerns prompted the Torah, or the Talmudic rabbis, to issue their restrictions. Rather, the laws of *kashrut* provide a discipline for Jewish living.

The Jewish life cycle consists of rituals which guide the Jew from the cradle to beyond the grave. Eight days after birth, a male Jewish child is entered into the covenant of Abraham through the procedure of circumcision (*brit milah*, "covenant of circumcision") at which the foreskin of the penis is surgically removed. Traditionally, a trained circumciser (*mohel*) would conduct the ritual in the home or in the synagogue, though today some parents opt to have the procedure performed in the hospital by a physician. At age 13, the ceremony of Bar or Bat Mitzvah ("son or daughter of the commandment") is conducted, at which the child leads the synagogue in worship and reads the Torah in Hebrew, demonstrating a competence in Jewish life. The final life cycle portal is death, on which more is addressed below.

Lastly, there are two values which underlie and influence core Jewish practices: a commitment to cleanliness and a duty to modesty. By *halacha* (Jewish law), the Jew is required to wash one's hands at least seven times daily, including in the morning upon awakening, before eating, and upon touching any matter which is considered unclean. In the year 1348, for instance, when the Black Death pandemic devastated Europe with the bubonic plague, killing up to 50 percent of the general populace, the plague's incidence in Jewish communities was only a fraction of that elsewhere because Jews washed their hands regularly, thus defeating the spread of the disease. (Ironically, to explain how Jews were lesser affected by the plague, calumnious charges were propagated that Jews had caused the outbreak by poisoning the wells. Widespread oppression of Jews resulted.) Modesty (*tzniyut*) especially guides interaction between genders, principally in the Orthodox community. Among the Orthodox who are most observant of *halacha*, unmarried men and women do not touch, and a married man is not to touch or have any contact with women other than those of his immediate family. This limitation may cause Jewish women to seek female care providers when seeking medical treatment, though this would be suspended in life-threatening situations because of *piku'ah nefesh*. As well, among those who are observant of *halacha*, a woman will not have sexual relations with her husband while she is menstruating and is ritually unclean, and for one week thereafter.

Health and disease

Central to health beliefs within Judaism is that the body is a vessel which is a gift from God and is not to be violated. As such, the corollary also is true: that the physician has an obligation to heal and to return the condition of health to the ailing patient. Maimonides, the medieval Jewish physician and philosopher, taught in his code of Jewish law that the physician who withholds his services is considered as shedding blood (*Yoreh De'ah* 336:1). This duty is derived from the biblical command, "You shall love your neighbor as yourself" (Leviticus 19:18). Yet, there is a theological conflict which arises from this charge to engage in the human art of healing. Namely, should one posit that all health and illnesses are ultimately derived from God, who is the source of life and of the natural order of the universe, the physician's intercession on behalf of healing represents a contravention and even an indictment of the divine system. By what right may the healthcare provider apply knowledge and skill and potentially breach the normal flow of health and illness? The Talmudic rabbis struggled with this concept, yet argued that just as the soap maker creates soap to facilitate cleaning and the farmer uses fertilizer to stimulate plant growth, so too a physician may employ the healing arts to engender healing. "Drugs and medicaments are the fertilizer and the physician is the tiller of the soil" (Eisenstein 1915: 581).

An early health belief which governed biblical practices was a profound regard for blood and bodily fluids. The Torah regarded blood as the life source and life force of both human and animal beings. Thus, among the laws of *kashrut* is the removal of blood from meat (see Leviticus 17:10, 19:26). For human health, the ancient priest was to inspect bodily discharges and skin ailments for discoloration, and a person with such a discharge was rendered impure and sequestered until he was deemed fit to be readmitted. Though greatly discussed in the Torah, these matters no longer govern modern Jewish life.

As described above, although circumcision, regard for cleanliness and modesty, and attention to *kashrut* are each general Judaic practices, each also may be construed as health practices. Circumcision certainly requires the trained hand of the circumciser, use of the proper implements, respect for cleanliness in healing, and the sensitive care of family to palliate the attendant suffering of the week-old infant. Although circumcision is a ritual practice, it surely is one of the earliest prescribed and regulated surgical procedures in human society, dating back to the patriarchal period (early to mid-second millennium BCE). Cleanliness, though initially charged as a social and ritual concern, may also be understood today as a matter of personal and social hygiene. Similarly, insofar as modesty unwittingly regulates human contact, it also may serve a social hygiene consideration by limiting the transfer of disease. Lastly, *kashrut* originally served to differentiate the Jewish community from others and to provide discipline to Jewish daily life. That later research would demonstrate that many proscribed animals also carry disease or uncleanness adds a health element to this otherwise basic routine.

Among the principal commandments in Judaism is *bikur cholim* (visiting the sick). Although not expressly commanded in the Torah, the law is derived by the Talmudic rabbis from God visiting Abraham in the days following the patriarch's self-administered circumcision at the age of 99 (Genesis 17:24, 18:1). The Talmud states, "As God clothes the naked, you clothe the naked. The Holy One visits the sick, as it is written, 'And God appeared to him (Abraham); so you visit the sick'" (BT *Sotah* 14a). Visiting the sick acts as a restorative, the rabbis taught. As God has implanted within every human being the image of God, which illness subverts, the visitor at the bedside reaffirms that divine value. Two thousand years ago, "Rabbi Acha bar Chanina taught, 'Whoever visits a sick person takes away one-sixtieth of his suffering'" (BT *Nedarim* 39b). Elsewhere in the Talmud, *bikur cholim* is considered one of the ten chief ethical commandments, the fulfillment of which is unlimited, and which yields fruit for all eternity (BT *Shabbat* 127a).

Lastly, within consideration of health practices it is worthy to note that Jewish teachings regarding sexual behavior and sexual mores affect both communal and individual health. In its table of prohibited relations, the Torah forbids marital and thus sexual unions between close members of the family (Leviticus 18). Surely, the Torah was unaware of genetic science and the risk of an overly homogeneous genetic pool on the healthy diversity of the population. Proscribed unions likely were banned out of a sense of social morality and family probity. Yet, this also served to diversify the gene pool in an early stage of social development, thus promoting healthier progeny. Procreation clearly is the intent of sexual relations in the Torah, as evidenced in God's first communication to Adam, "Be fruitful and multiply" (Genesis 1:28). Later, Maimonides would add the elements of pleasure and fulfillment as benefits of sexuality. Regulations, however, governed the sexual instinct. The woman was restricted from coitus while menstruating, and the Torah forbade the destruction of male seed – hence, male masturbation. Talmudic and later rabbinic commentators deliberated over permitted and prohibited means of contraception, though it is clear from the Talmud that contraception itself was allowed, and even required in certain circumstances. A nursing mother, for instance, must refrain from conceiving lest she wean her child prematurely, resulting in death (BT *Yebamot* 12b). Today, there are differences of opinion regarding the use of contraceptives within the Orthodox Jewish community, as precoital and postcoital devices may waste or destroy semen, thus conflicting with the prohibition. For all Jews, and especially more observant Jews, the use of oral contraceptives is less objectionable on *halachic* grounds and is even referenced in the Talmud when the wife of an early rabbi used a potion to render her sterile (BT *Yevamot* 65b). Currently, birth control procedures are commonplace in the Jewish community, except among the ultra-Orthodox.

There are a number of diseases which, in the Jewish community, are commonly known as "Jewish genetic diseases," including Tay-Sachs disease, Gaucher disease type 1, Bloom's disease, familial dysautonomia, cystic fibrosis, and more recently breast and ovarian cancer. These illnesses appear in subsets of the Jewish community far more prevalently than in the general population and are recognized as genetic disorders occurring in Ashkenazic Jewish families from Eastern Europe. Due to social and religious conditions which prevailed for many centuries, the genetic mutations which resulted in these diseases became concentrated in this population, such that presently one in five Ashkenazic Jews may be a carrier of a gene for a threatening condition, according to the Jewish Genetic Disease Consortium. Today, many Jewish couples are encouraged to undergo genetic screening prior to marriage to determine if they are carriers of a mutation, and, if they are carriers, to consider amniocentesis and fetal monitoring during potential pregnancy.

Recent studies also have shown that the genetic mutations known as BRCA1 and BRCA2, which predispose one toward hereditary breast or ovarian cancer, also occur inordinately in Ashkenazic Jewish women. For Jewish women who carry BRCA1, the mutation accounts for 16 percent of breast cancers and 39 percent of ovarian cancers, compared with 4 percent and 12 percent, respectively, in the general population. Moreover, in families with a history of breast or ovarian cancer, those in the Jewish community who carry the mutation have an 80–90 percent lifetime risk of breast cancer and a 40–50 percent lifetime risk of ovarian cancer. These data raise significant ethical and medical considerations, including concerns for prophylactic mastectomies, potential curative genetic engineering, insurability, and the welfare of one's children or grandchildren (Dorff 2003: 156; Rosner and Bleich 1987: 178; Bleich 1981: 103; Ford et al. 1994: 692–695; Struewing et al. 1995: 198–200; Kohn 2008: 14–21).

Turning to some prominent bioethical issues that impact all religions, Jewish tradition views life as beginning at birth – when the first breath of the newborn is inhaled. Life does not begin at conception. In fact, the Hebrew word for "soul" and for "breathing" are linked, *nefesh*, demonstrating that a soul is a breathing being. Thus, in the discussion regarding abortion, Judaism bears a distinct religious position. It asserts that since life commences with the newly-born infant breathing independently of the mother, then abortion represents feticide – the destruction of a fetus – not infanticide, the killing of a human child's life. Yet, in the millennia of Jewish life, there have been varying opinions.

The Torah describes an incident in which a miscarriage occurs:

> When men fight, and one of them pushes a pregnant woman and a miscarriage results, but no other damage ensues, the one responsible shall be fined according as the woman's husband may exact from him, the payment to be based on reckoning.
>
> (Exodus 21:22)

This verse demonstrates that Torah considers the loss of a fetus not to be a capital offense. Potential life is not equivalent to an actual life. Rather, the fetus is considered as any other body part of the woman which may suffer injury in an accident, and for which pecuniary compensation for damages is determined by a judge. Later rabbinic interpretation in the Mishnah (*Oholot* 7:6) affirmed that the life of the mother takes precedence over that of the fetus. This was further confirmed by Maimonides in his code of Jewish law (*Hilchot Rotzeach* 1:9), though Maimonides added a caveat that the fetus may be destroyed because it is equivalent to an aggressor (*rodef*) which pursues and threatens the mother. Elsewhere, Jewish law details parameters of the *rodef*, delimiting the privileges of one who is threatened and respecting certain rights even of the aggressor. For instance, a homeowner at night may defend the family against an intruder and use deadly force assuming that the *rodef* is armed. However, during daylight the homeowner is not allowed to use such force unless the severity of the threat can be verified. Applying this line of Jewish legal reasoning, a pregnant woman may only abort the fetus when the pregnancy represents a significant danger to her life or well-being. Unresolved in Jewish thought are the limits to that threat: Is psychological or economic peril sufficient to justify abortion? Must there be a threat to life, or may it constitute a danger to the woman's well-being? These questions have not been decided definitively and are left to each individual's perspective on Judaism and ethics. There are those, especially in the Orthodox community, who argue that all forms of human life are sacred, including that in a test tube. Hence, they oppose all but necessary therapeutic abortions as infanticide. In the Progressive Jewish communities, the common interpretation is that the woman's rights take precedence over those of the potential life of the fetus and that abortion is a personal choice.

Regarding euthanasia and physician-assisted suicide, Judaism begins with the conviction, above all, that life is sacred. It is a gift from God and actually does not belong to human beings. Rather, humans are stewards of the life which is given. However, in the Mishnah, the rabbis taught, "Against your will you live, and against your will you die" (*Avot* 4:22). Yet, how much will is one free to exercise over the timeframes of one's life? When the conditions of life include exceptionally difficult suffering, may one choose to terminate life? Moreover, heeding the dictum of Ecclesiastes, which teaches that there is naturally, by divine design, "a time for being born and a time for dying" (Ecclesiastes 3:2), may one self-arrogate the decision as to when is the "time for dying"? Conversely, when it appears that the time for dying is nigh, may one hasten that time, or remove impediments which are sustaining life and thereby preventing the time for dying from asserting itself?

Judaism recognizes that there are two varieties of euthanasia, active and passive. Active euthanasia is an unjustified form of killing and is prohibited. Passive euthanasia, however, raises further questions. Modern medical technology can greatly prolong the life of a dying person and even sustain one who otherwise would have died. Is it permissible by Jewish teachings to disconnect that apparatus and to allow the person to expire naturally? Or is one duty-bound to undertake all measures, even extreme, to protect and prolong life?

The story of the death of an exalted sage of the Mishnah is illustrative. The sage, called "Rabbi" due to his lofty standing, was dying, and his disciples gathered around his bedside to pray that God would allow Rabbi further life. Seeing that her master was suffering and agitated by the prayers of his students, Rabbi's handmaid threw an earthen jug to the ground where it burst with a great noise. The disciples were startled and momentarily ceased their prayers. In that quiet instant, Rabbi's soul departed (BT *Ketubot* 104a). Interestingly, the Talmud does not censure the handmaid, but rather authorizes the episode.

This vignette offers an early example of passive euthanasia. Rabbi was dying, and the prayers of his students were comparable to life-support equipment in a modern hospital; they were an impediment to Rabbi's dying process. The maid opted to "unplug" the equipment and to allow Rabbi to die. The death of Rabbi, arguably the Mishnah's greatest figure, serves to validate passive euthanasia. Yet it also sets conditions for its permissibility. Judaism forbids any directly euthanizing action which prompts death, but for the *goses* (moribund patient) it sets no obligation to continue treatment or to prolong life. As such, removal of artificial nutrition or hydration is treated similarly, as it allows the course of death to continue. As well, quality of life is not the determining factor. The death of Rabbi occurred not to palliate a quality of life concern, but rather to remove an impediment to an imminent death.

The question of physician-assisted suicide follows similar reasoning. The physician is charged with prolonging life as well as with finding cures. Any action which actively hastens death is unjustifiable, yet should death be looming, the physician is not obliged to extend life. However, what of the case of a man who is suffering so mightily that he cries out, "Let me die!" May the physician heed his demands and assist him in ending his life? Jewish law also forbids suicide and treats it as unjustified killing (though to mitigate the anguish on mourners, the rabbis determined to treat suicide as an accident). Assisting one to commit suicide, therefore, is the same as abetting a murder and is not allowed. Clearly, however, physicians are stirred by the compelling moral desire to mollify pain and bring comfort to suffering patients. Jewish law does not prohibit a physician from prescribing strong analgesic medications such as morphine to control pain yet which may concurrently suppress respiratory function and allow the process of dying to proceed. Palliative care is understood in Judaism as proper and necessary, yet it must be managed carefully when death is near. In 1997, the Conservative Movement's Committee on Jewish Law and Standards issued a ruling which stated, "Patients and their caregivers ... have the tradition's permission to withhold or withdraw impediments to the natural process of dying..." (Dorff 2003: 376).

When it comes to gender relations, Judaism makes no distinction either in the value of life or in treatment based on the gender of the patient. All life is of equal value. Similarly, there is no gender limitation as to who may work in healthcare fields. Of concern regarding gender, as discussed above, is regard for *tzniyut* (modesty). Primarily in the Orthodox community, women must have the option to see female healthcare providers so as not to risk violating this precept.

Death and dying

In the Book of Ecclesiastes one reads the famous poem, "A season is set for everything, a time for every experience under heaven: A time for being born and a time for dying" (Ecclesiastes 3:1–2). Death, therefore, is considered a natural part of the flow of life, and certainly in earlier days it was a regular experience of adults and children alike. The Torah records that, upon death, each of the patriarchs "was gathered to his kin" (Genesis 25:17, 35:29, 49:33). Natural death occurred in the family chambers, not in hospitals or nursing facilities where today death is moderated, mitigated, and euphemized. Thus, in understanding and respecting death and treating it as the portal to the great mystery of beyond, Judaism also imbued death and dying with very practical, intimate, and earthly boundaries and protocols.

A near-death person is called a *goses* (moribund). This is not a medically technical definition, but rather defines the patient who is in a persistent and deteriorating non-responsive condition. This description heralds the expected close of life. In Jewish tradition, life begins at the first breath in accordance with the second creation story in Genesis. Describing the creation of man in the Garden of Eden, Torah recounts, "He (God) blew into his nostrils the breath of life, and man became a living being" (Genesis 2:7). As such, classical Jewish thinking held that life's parameters begin and end with breathing – when the soul enters and departs from the body. Thus, death occurs with the cessation of breathing. The rabbis prescribe taking much care to be certain that breathing has ceased and that death has occurred, even waiting half an hour before removing the body from the deathbed. Liturgically, it is a custom that the dying person, or a surrogate if not capable, recites a final prayer of forgiveness as death approaches.

Because Jewish funeral procedures were designed in the ancient Near East in days before refrigeration and because Jewish law prohibits defacing the body (hence, disallowing embalming), burial was to occur expeditiously once death is confirmed – that is, within 24 hours, if possible. Thus, today there may be pressure on the physician to swiftly complete the necessary certification to allow the family and the funeral professionals to arrange for a timely burial. Respecting Jewish law, which dictates that the body is a sacred vessel of life, the body is not to be left alone. Observant Jews will arrange for a *shomeir* (a watchman) to sit with the body in the funeral establishment until it is prepared for burial and to recite words of the Psalms. As well, in keeping with tradition of not disfiguring the body, cremation was disallowed, although today some will opt for cremation. Historically, for the same reasons, autopsies were prohibited, except where municipal statutes require them.

Similarly, organ transplantation presented significant difficulties. *Piku'ah nefesh*, the primacy of saving a life, allows one to suspend or violate most Jewish laws in order to save a life. Yet, in the early days of organ transplantation, the procedure often resulted in both the death of the donor and defacing the donor's body. Thus, in the 1960s, rabbinic authorities determined that transplantation risked greater hazards than were allowed and concluded that organ transplantation was tantamount to murder, thus was not permissible. Only with new drugs which suppressed the immune system, granting the recipient a realistic chance at survival, did the leading Orthodox medical ethicists consent to organ transplantation. Presently, motivated by the Jewish ethics of fixing the world and saving lives, many synagogues conduct donor promotions, encouraging congregants to register as potential donors.

The Jewish funeral is not theological. Its primary purpose is to guide and support the mourners to manage their difficult process of grieving and balancing their lives anew, rather than to usher the soul of the deceased into eternity. Admittedly, the mystery of what is beyond death compels the Jew and the non-Jew alike, yet Judaism is steeped in commandments which guide the Jew to live in the present world. Thus, the Jewish funeral is often brief and relatively lacking in pageantry. Sharing memories and expressing care for the bereaved are the central components of the funeral.

Conclusion

Judaism, and Jews, have a long history and regard for health and healing. Similarly, Jewish sacred texts and *halacha*, Jewish law, include much instruction addressing practice and values which govern medical behavior and ethics. Originating in the Hebrew Bible and continuing through each successive stratum of Jewish legal literature, including the Mishnah, Talmud, and codes of the great philosophers and codifiers such as Moses Maimonides, central precepts such as the sanctity of life and respect for

Table 10.1 Dos and don'ts

Dos	Don'ts
1 Be sensitive to the Jewish festival calendar and holy days which have specific expectations or limitations. 2 Be respectful of the dietary concerns of *kashrut*. Besides making available kosher foods for the hospitalized Jewish patient, awareness of particular dietary considerations due to festival customs also would be advised. 3 It is always encouraged that a rabbi or Jewish chaplain, where available, be informed when a Jewish patient is in the hospital.	1 One should kindly refrain from offering "theological explanations" of death to a bereaved Jewish family member. 2 One ought to be careful in touching – even offering a courtesy handshake – to an Orthodox Jew of the opposite gender. Thus, medically unnecessary contact ought to be resisted, and one should not be insulted if, when offering a handshake as an introduction in a hospital room, it is not accepted, or is rebuffed. 3 Be careful not to assume that a Jewish patient is either Orthodox or not Orthodox merely by his or her appearance. It may be wise to inquire if there are any religious considerations to be respected.

the body have always informed Jewish life and stimulated great attention to the healing arts. Thus, healthcare considerations are not secondary or tertiary within the Jewish religious system; rather they bear a central position in Judaism and compel basic ethics. Witness the inordinate number of Jews in the healing professions, which has been evident in every generation and in every region wherever Jews have resided. And, despite vast diversity in religious beliefs among adherents of different streams of Judaism, the Jewish world has built largely progressive positions on controversial ethical matters such as abortion, euthanasia, and organ transplantation. These positions are based on consideration for existent life over potential life, concern for the dignity of the patient, and most importantly, the primary ethos of saving life at all costs. Furthermore, in raising behaviors such as diet, cleanliness, and modesty to religious precepts, Judaism also instituted social hygiene as a sacred principle. In all, healthcare considerations are basic and fundamental to Judaism and to the Jewish people.

Case study

A 30-something African American couple brought their 14-year-old son to the Emergency Room for general malaise.

As the clinical ethicist, I received a call from one of the ER team because the physician had faced off against the parents in a combative, adversarial manner. According to the physician, the child needed a blood transfusion but the parents refused to consent to it. He told the parents it did not matter what their issues might be with regard to blood transfusions, their child was going to get transfused. The parents identified themselves as Jewish. With some internal conflict, being influenced by stereotypes, I thought to myself, "It is a bit unusual for African Americans to be Jewish." A further complicating matter is that most Jewish persons have no qualms about receiving blood transfusions. This is a common element of care for Jehovah's Witness families, but not Jewish families; at least not to my knowledge. But this is America and we can believe in and practice, pretty much, any religion we wish. In the process of this case, I learned a good deal about Hebrew Israelites, Black Hebrew Israelites, and Black Jews. Though not typically accepted as "Jewish" by the followers of Judaism, these groups do self-identify as directly related to the Jewish people of the Hebrew Bible.

The 14-year-old child was diagnosed with sickle cell anemia, a disease that is more prevalent in the African American community than in other ethnic groups. And while blood transfusions are a typical element of treatment for sickle cell patients, the hospital care team never did transfuse the child. As it turns out, the physician group that covered the Emergency Room is on contract with the hospital and the reality of the situation was that the patient–physician relationship was not exactly a concern of the physician group covering the ER. The hospital, of course, was very concerned for their effort to provide patient-centered care, but the physician was just filling his spot in the schedule. Thus, he appeared to the parents and the hospital staff as though he did not care at all about the parents and their religious desires for their child.

Questions for reflection

1   How do we manage the influence of our stereotypes when we face real people who do not fit into the normal categories? Should we talk about it with those we are caring for? Or just stick to the medical information?
2   Are some physicians or physician groups really so uncaring about what patients and their families want? Is the role of ER physicians to just technically care for the medical condition of their patients and not worry themselves about other aspects of their care?
3   What can/should hospitals do to make sure the physicians they contract with behave in ways consistent with the hospital's mission and values?

Glossary

Cantor or Hazzan   The Cantor is the officient who sings the Jewish liturgy during worship.

Erev Shabbat   This term refers to the time on Friday evening just prior to sunset when the Sabbath is about to begin.

Fleischig   The Yiddish term used to describe a meat-based meal.

Milchig   The Yiddish term used to describe a dairy-based meal.

Parve   The Yiddish term used to describe a meal which is neutral, neither dairy nor meat.

Rabbi or Rav   The terms used to refer to the religious leader of Jews.

Shabbat or Shabbes   The Sabbath Day, Saturday.

Siddur   The Jewish prayer book.

Synagogue, Temple or Shul   The facility or building of Jewish worship and study.

Torah   The scroll of the Five Books of Moses.

Bibliography

Bleich, J. D. (1981) *Judaism and Healing: Halachic Perspectives*, New York: Ktav Publishing House.

Della Pergola, S. (2010) *World Jewish Population, 2010* (Rep.), North American Jewish Data Bank.

Dorff, E. N. (2003) *Matters of Life and Death: A Jewish Approach to Modern Medical Ethics*, Philadelphia: The Jewish Publication Society.

Eisenstein, J. D. (ed.) (1915) *Otzar Midrashim*, vol. 2, New York: Mishor.

Ford, D., Easton, D. F., Bishop, D. T., Narod, S. A., and Goldgar, D. E. (1994) "Risks of cancer in BRCA1-mutation carriers," *Lancet*, vol. 343: 692–695.

Greenberg, S. and Levine, J. D. (eds) (1978) *Mahzor Chadash: The New Mahzor*, Bridgeport, CT: Media Judaica.

Kohn, D. J. (ed.) (2008) *Life, Faith, and Cancer: Jewish Journeys Through Diagnosis, Treatment, and Recovery*, New York: URJ Press.

Rosner, F. and Bleich, J. D. (eds) (1987) *Jewish Bioethics*, New York: Hebrew Publishing.

Struewing, J. P., Abeliovich, D., Perez, T., Avishai, N., Kaback, M. M., Collins, F. S., and Brody, L. C. (1995) "The carrier frequency of the BRCA1 185delAG mutation is approximately 1 percent in Ashkenazi Jewish individuals," *Nature Genetics*, vol. 11: 198–200.

United Jewish Communities: The Federations of North America (2001) "National Jewish Population Survey 2000–01." Available online at: www.jewishdatabank. org/studies/details.cfm?StudyID=307 (accessed September 29, 2016).

Suggested texts

Bleich, J. D. (1981) *Judaism and Healing: Halachic Perspectives*, New York: Ktav Publishing House.

Dorff, E. N. (2003) *Matters of Life and Death: A Jewish Approach to Modern Medical Ethics*, Philadelphia: The Jewish Publication Society.

Rosner, F. (2006) *Contemporary Biomedical Ethical Issues and Jewish Law*, Jersey City, NJ: Ktav Publishing House.

Rosner, F. and Bleich, J. D. (eds) (1987) *Jewish Bioethics*, New York: Hebrew Publishing.

Weintraub, S. Y. (ed.) (1994) *Healing of Soul, Healing of Body*, Woodstock, VT: Jewish Lights.

11 Christianity

David R. Larson

For God so loved the world that he gave his only son, so that everyone who
believes in him may not perish but have eternal life.

Jesus Christ

He said to him, "you shall love the Lord your God with all your heart, and
with all your soul, and with all your mind." This is the greatest and first
commandment. And a second is like it: "You shall love your neighbor as
yourself." On these two commandments hang all the law and the prophets.

Jesus Christ

Introduction

With more than two billion adherents, Christianity is the largest and most
widely dispersed religion in the world today. It is also very diverse, especially in what it says and does about health and healing. On the one hand,
as evidenced by the pilgrimages to places like Lourdes in France, where
millions of Christians have gone each year for generations in quest of
miraculous cures, or as seen more controversially in movies like *Elmer
Gantry* and *Leap of Faith*, its healing methods can be simple, unsophisti-
cated, and sometimes even superstitious. On the other hand, over the centuries and in our own time, virtually everywhere Christians have gone they
have established some of the best hospitals and universities in the effort to
help humankind deal with illness and disease.

Some may find it difficult to see much similarity between "faith healing"
meetings before huge numbers of awe-struck people gathered in public
places like gymnasiums, stadiums, and huge tents, on the one hand, and
the quiet scientific activity of Christian institutions that treat sick people
with resources such as chemotherapy, organ transplantation, and proton
beam accelerators. These differences are real and significant. But for better
or for worse, they are all part of the Christian story.

Demographics

Beginning with Italy and moving north and west, most Christians in Europe adhere to Roman Catholicism, the largest of the three primary branches of Christianity. So do those in Quebec in Canada and many in the southwestern portions of the United States. The whole of South America and virtually all of the Philippines are also Roman Catholic.

Protestants in Western Europe are most numerous in portions of Germany, all of Scandinavia and the United Kingdom. They are also the primary Christian populations in North America, Australia, New Zealand, and South Africa. Protestants take second place in overall numbers worldwide to Roman Catholics. Both are exploding numerically in Africa south of the Sahara Desert.

Starting with Greece and moving roughly north until reaching Russia and then turning sharply east, and covering the vast expanse from there and all the way to the Pacific Ocean, Christians lean toward Eastern Orthodoxy. It is the smallest of the three primary branches of Christianity in numbers.

All told, Christians in the United States comprise about 70.6 percent of the population. Approximately 20.8 percent of the total population is Roman Catholic. They are rather evenly spread throughout the different regions of the country (Wormald 2015).

Approximately 26 percent of the nation's total population is Evangelical (conservative) Protestant. The largest number of these is Baptist of one sort or another (15.4 percent). In significantly smaller numbers, there are the Nondenominational (6.2 percent), Pentecostals (4.6 percent), and Lutheran Evangelicals (3.5 percent). The other groups of Evangelical Christians are dispersed among 15 or so smaller groups. The greatest number of Evangelical Protestants lives in the South and Midwest (Wormald 2015).

About 14.7 percent of the people in the United States are Mainline (liberal) Protestants. The most numerous of these are Methodist (3.9 percent). The Lutherans and the Baptists are the next largest groups and each comprises 2.1 percent of the population. Those with non-specific affiliations comprise 1.9 percent, while Episcopalians make up 1.4 percent. The remaining 4 percent or so of Mainline Protestants can be found in smaller groups. The Mainline Protestants have their greatest numbers in the South and Midwest. Almost 7 percent of all Americans belong to Historically Black Protestant Churches. Most of these are Baptists (4 percent). The others (about 2.5 percent) are in smaller groups. Like the Evangelical Protestants, they are active mostly in the South and West (Wormald 2015).

History

Born in Bethlehem and reared in Nazareth, as Christians remember it, Jesus left his carpenter shop as a young man and became a traveling preacher, teacher, and healer. His message was that the Kingdom or Reign of God was at hand and that in some ways it was already present. Like the Hebrew scriptures he had studied, he taught that true morality can be summarized in love for God and neighbor. Yet he emphasized the need for a way of life that was more inward, thoroughgoing, and inclusive.

Some political and religious leaders of the time took offense at Jesus' words and deeds, interpreting his emphasis upon God's Kingdom or Reign as a threat to their own. This is why Pontius Pilate, the primary representative of the Roman Empire which was occupying the land, had him tortured and then killed by crucifixion. Most Christians believe that on the third day after his death he was resurrected. After a brief time he ascended to heaven with a promise someday soon to return in power and glory.

The first 500 years of Christian history were marked by rapid growth and increasing cultural influence. Emperor Constantine made Christianity the official religion of the Roman Empire in 323 CE. The first eight Ecumenical Councils (large and sometimes lengthy meetings of Christian leaders designed to bring consistency to Christian theology and teachings) took place between the fourth and ninth centuries. The Council of Nicaea formulated the most frequently recited Christian creed:

> I believe in one God, the Father Almighty, Maker of heaven and earth, and of all things visible and invisible. And in one Lord Jesus Christ, the only-begotten Son of God, begotten of the Father before all worlds; God of God, Light of Light, very God of very God; begotten, not made, being of one substance with the Father, by whom all things were made. Who, for us men and for our salvation, came down from heaven, and was incarnate by the Holy Spirit of the virgin Mary, and was made man; and was crucified also for us under Pontius Pilate; He suffered and was buried; and the third day He rose again, according to the Scriptures; and ascended into heaven, and sits on the right hand of the Father; and He shall come again, with glory, to judge the quick and the dead; whose kingdom shall have no end. And I believe in the Holy Ghost, the Lord and Giver of Life; who proceeds from the Father and the Son; who with the Father and the Son together is worshipped and glorified; who spoke by the prophets. And I believe one holy catholic and apostolic Church. I acknowledge one baptism for the remission of sins; and I look for the resurrection of the dead, and the life of the world to come. Amen.
>
> (Nicene Creed 325 CE)

Roman Catholicism dominated in Western Europe for centuries, with the theologian Augustine of North Africa in the fifth century and Thomas Aquinas in Italy and France in the thirteenth century as the era's intellectual giants. Orthodoxy was far more influential in the Eastern part of the Roman Empire, a split that remains into the twenty-first century.

History began to move away from Rome beginning with the Renaissance in fourteenth-century Italy. Tensions boiled over with the Protestant Reformation in the sixteenth century, preeminently with Martin Luther in Germany and John Calvin in Switzerland. Against what they perceived to be spiritual and administrative abuses of the church, the reformers emphasized the authority of Scripture – as interpreted by individual Christians – over against that of the church hierarchy, the centrality of salvation by God's grace (without any human participation), and the "priesthood" of all believers – that every Christian has received a calling from God for ministry and each calling is equally sacred.

The seventeenth century in Western Europe was beset by religious warfare. This contributed to the flowering of the European Enlightenment, which triggered the switch from pre-modern to modern ways of thinking and acting. One response, deism with its naturalistic view of God and the universe, eliminated much of Christianity in the name of human reason. This was the religion of Thomas Jefferson, Benjamin Franklin, and other American leaders. A second response was the Evangelical Revival in England and North America. Its leaders – principally John and Charles Wesley and George Whitefield from England and Jonathan Edwards in America – put more emphasis upon emotion, what Edwards called "the religious affections" (Edwards 1959).

Many positive things occurred in the nineteenth century, such as the largest missionary endeavors in Christian history, the elimination of slavery even in North America and the United Kingdom, and the establishment of many Christian voluntary service societies. But the American Civil War, fought primarily by Christians, cut an ugly wound. Also, with the findings of Charles Darwin, Karl Marx, Sigmund Freud, and many others, Christianity's conceptual foundations began to quake. World War I dashed the hopes for an era of unprecedented peace and prosperity. The modern era had ended and the postmodern one had begun.

These challenges flowed into the twentieth century. Some, embracing modernism, sought to integrate newer scientific findings with their Christian beliefs; others, who objected, moved in the direction now referred to as fundamentalism. This divide has sliced across Christian denominations in America as well as between them into the twenty-first century.

At the end of the twentieth century, Roman Catholicism, which had assimilated enough to see one of its own, John F. Kennedy, become president of the United States, and Evangelical Protestantism, which had done the same thing at least twice, in Jimmy Carter and George W. Bush, amounted to the most vibrant forms of Christianity in the United States.

Throughout its long history, Christianity has made many contributions to theoretical and practical medicine – beginning with Eastern Orthodoxy's introduction of the first hospitals. Yet it is impossible to list all of these because it is difficult to distinguish the history of Western medicine from the history of Western Judaism, Christianity, and Islam. Although these are somewhat different streams, their waters intermingle so often and so deeply that it is not easy to specifically distinguish where one begins and the other ends. What is more, the greatest contributions of these religions to health and healing may have been more philosophical and theological.

Beliefs and practices

General

Christian beliefs differ greatly in their details; however, if one stands back and considers them from a distance, they appear remarkably similar in their main outlines. Also, Christians share many convictions with Jews and Muslims. All three are "Abrahamic" religions because they each recount their formative narrative to the person and faith of the biblical personage, Abraham.

Like Jews and Muslims, Christians center their lives on the one true God who brought the universe into being and continues to sustain it. God is both immanent, within the universe, and transcendent, beyond and greater than it. There is no place where God is absent, nothing that can be known that God does not know and nothing that can be done that God cannot do. Everything about God is worthy of admiration and acclaim. This is especially so of God's steadfast love that endures forever.

Most Christians believe that the one genuine God is "Triune." As many early Christians put it, "the one God exists in three Persons and one substance, Father, Son, and Holy Spirit." The word "substance" means "essence." The word "person" comes from the different masks or roles of actors in theatrical performances. "Perichoresis," or "dancing in a circle," instead of vertically or horizontally, is one metaphor Christians have used when thinking about the three members of the Trinity. One implication of this doctrine is that relationships characterize everything, from God to subatomic particles and smaller.

Although they vary in their emphasis, Christians believe that God is revealed in nature, history, experience, reason, scripture, and, most decisively, in Jesus Christ. Like Jews and Muslims, Christians are "people of the book." This book, the "Bible," is actually a "library" with material from many different times and places. Taken together, these documents from long ago tell a story. It is a story about God's interaction with people and other things. Christians believe that this story points the direction in which our lives should move today.

The biblical idea of creation distinguishes Christian belief from at least two other alternatives. One of them is the kind of dualism that posits a deep, wide, and unbridgeable divide between the spiritual and physical realms of human life; the second is the kind of monism or pantheism that pictures the universe as a single whole, with all particular things and people as its partial expressions. Christians believe that dualism is too negative about the physical features of life and that monism or pantheism undervalues the relative individuality of each thing.

Christians believe that all human beings are created in the "image of God," the expression coming from the biblical account of the creation of humankind. This does not mean that they look like God. It means that they share in a limited and imperfect way some of God's most important characteristics: reason, freedom, memory, anticipation, purposefulness, intimacy, and perhaps even laughter. Although other animals possess these characteristics in lesser or greater degrees, they characterize human life in a qualitatively superior way.

The basic idea of the Christian concept of sin is that pain, suffering, and evil are not essential elements of existence. "Intruders" and "violators," they are the global consequences of misusing the freedom God has given humankind. "Original sin" refers to the difficulties and inabilities all people inherit. "Actual sins" are the thoughts, words, and deeds in which they freely indulge even when they know they should not. Christians believe that everyone except Jesus Christ is a sinner.

They believe that human beings cannot extricate themselves from sin and its consequences: discord, guilt, meaninglessness, and death. This is something only God can do. The entire Bible is a story of how God has repeatedly done this for others and the assurance that God can do the same for people today. All religions have a story. For many of them, it is explanatory; for Christians it is essential. They believe that the story of salvation is the best of all narratives because it proclaims the good news that God loves unconditionally.

The word "Jesus" is a name, the word "Christ" a title. It conveys the meaning of the prior Hebrew words: "Messiah" or "Anointed." For Christians, Jesus Christ is the long-awaited Jewish "Messiah." He is "Immanuel," which is to say, "God with Us," when the word "Us" refers to everybody; all of humankind.

Christians believe that Jesus Christ was the incarnation of God, the embodiment of God in human life. In this sense, Jesus was truly human and truly God. When Christians talk of Jesus as the "Son of God" they do not mean that their relationship was like the biological one between human fathers and sons. They are speaking as the ancients did when describing God's reaction to the coronation of a new King. "This is my beloved son," or "This is my only begotten son," God said in praise of the new monarch. According to the Biblical story, this is what God said of Jesus.

From the very start it has been difficult for Christians to avoid confusion in their two-fold conviction that Jesus was truly God and truly man. One of the earliest problems was called "Docetism." It denied the true humanity of Jesus, holding that he only appeared to be human. "Arianism" eventually became a problem as well. It denied the true divinity of Jesus, picturing him as divine but not equal with God. There were many other similar challenges. In 451 CE, the Council of Chalcedon declared:

We confess that one and the same Christ, Lord, and only-begotten Son, is to be acknowledged in two natures without confusion, change, division, or separation. The distinction between natures was never abolished by their union, but rather the character proper to each of the two natures was preserved as they came together in one person and one hypostasis.

(Chalcedon 451 CE)

This settled the issue for most Christians, even if some have continued debating it ever since.

In addition to Jesus' preaching, teaching, and healing, most Christians emphasize his death and resurrection and their special importance in freeing humans from sin and its negative consequences: discord, guilt, meaninglessness, and death. In trying to explain how this happens they have used various analogies, as the Bible itself does, and each reflects the social settings from which it emerges.

Maybe the process of atonement is like being found guilty in a court of law and having someone else pay the penalty or take the punishment. Or perhaps it is like being kidnapped and then being set free because someone else paid the ransom. Or could it be that the process is more like a school in which we learn about God's love when we concentrate on the final hours of Jesus' life, seeing how he chose to accept suffering than to inflict it upon others? Christians have used all of these metaphors, and many others, claiming all along that the full process of atonement is beyond the capacity of mere words to describe.

Christians believe that the church is the "body of Christ," meaning that today it continues the preaching, teaching, and healing ministry of Jesus. Many apply it to Christians in all denominations; however, others restrict its usage to those they take to be genuine.

Christians differ in how they view the billions of people around the world who are not Christians. Many hold that these persons cannot experience salvation because they have not decided to become followers of Jesus, and this is so even if they have never heard of him. Many others hold that God is equally at work in all the religions of the world and that their genuine adherents are all equally saved. Most Christians take one of many alternatives between these extremes. One of these "middle" alternatives holds that, even though God is at work in all religions, people who are active in ones other than Christianity can still benefit from hearing its "good news," and that Christians can benefit from hearing theirs.

Christian worship and life center upon rituals or practices signifying the presence of God in ordinary life called "sacraments." Roman Catholic and Eastern Orthodox Christians hold that there are seven: (1) *baptism*, the use of water to celebrate the beginning of a new Christian life, (2) *confirmation*, determining on the basis of further consideration to live as a Christian, (3) *matrimony*, the lifelong, loving, and sexually exclusive union of a man and woman who establish a Christian home, (4) *penance*, doing sometimes difficult things that provide discipline when it is needed, (5) *prayer for the sick*, asking God for strength and wisdom in the face of illness and death, (6) *holy orders*, the decision by some to live their entire lives in service to the church as priests, and (7) *communion* or the Eucharist, a celebration with bread and wine as emblems of the sacrificial body and blood of Jesus Christ. Most Protestant Christians practice only two of the seven sacraments: baptism and communion.

Just as they believe that Jesus Christ was resurrected from the grave, the majority of Christians hold that they will experience life in the hereafter. But again they differ on the details. Most hold that the body and soul are so different that the soul does not die when the body does, and that instead the soul goes either to heaven, paradise, or to hell, punishment. Some contend that body and soul are inseparable, and that death includes the entire person, body and soul alike. They do not even like to talk about "body *and* soul," as though they are basically different. They much prefer "embodied soul" or "in-souled body," or just plain "person." Both groups look forward to the resurrection of the dead at the end of time when, according to one view, body and soul are reunited, or according to the other view, persons are given new life as integrated wholes.

Health and disease

Christians hold a positive view of the human body and its natural environment. Genuine wellbeing from this perspective is not about fleeing the material world in favor of the spiritual. Neither is it a matter of escaping individuality in union with the Whole or Absolute. Rather, it is the balanced integration and successful functioning of all aspects of life: physical, mental, social, ethical, and spiritual.

At least three types of disease flow from this understanding of health. The first is the malady of partiality. This occurs when an individual or society wholly disregards some important aspect of life, such as sex or spirituality. A second type of disease is the malady of imbalance and disintegration. Succeeding financially but not in other areas of life is an example. A third type of disease is the malady of unsuccessful functioning. This is what many people think of when they hear the word "disease." An eye that does not see, an ear that does not hear, or a brain that does not think are signs of ill health. This is the type of disease that medical professionals can most easily and effectively address.

Christians look at suffering – prolonged or continuing pain of any sort – in three primary ways. Some believe that God determines exactly what happens in every case, right down to the smallest detail. For them all suffering is good because everything fits into God's overall plan. Other Christians recoil at this suggestion. For them suffering is not good even though God can often help those who suffer to transform it into something good.

A third stance threads a path between the first two by distinguishing between existential (normal) and pathological (abnormal) types of suffering.

The suffering that parents often feel after all their children have moved is an example of the first. Trying to escape this kind of suffering is not wise. Suffering from a malignancy is an example of the second kind of suffering. According to this Christian stance, the second kind of suffering should be prevented or treated as aggressively as the first should be patiently endured.

Either pain or suffering that is not outweighed by its offsetting benefits is evil. Christians hold that this occurs in at least three ways. The first is *moral evil*. This is caused by the misuse of human freedom. Murdering a child is an obvious example. The second is *natural evil*, which occurs when something in the world of nature causes uncompensated pain or suffering. Tidal waves, earthquakes, and tornados are illustrations. The third, and by far the most difficult for many to contemplate, is *ecological evil*. This is the predatory nature of the whole of life, something most Christians see as a consequence of sin: nothing in this world lives without killing.

Many Christians acknowledge that the pervasiveness and apparent permanence of evil in its three forms is the single greatest challenge to Christian faith. This is because it is very difficult, both theoretically and experientially, to believe that the one true God is (1) wholly loving and (2) supremely powerful in light of (3) all the evil we observe and experience. This issue is often called the problem of "theodicy," a Greek word made up of two others that mean "God" and "righteousness" or "justice."

Christians today relate to theodicy, or the problem of evil and suffering in the world as it relates to God, in three primary ways. Some come close to denying that evil is real. They say that life is like a movie and that once we have come to its end we will see that every scene was necessary. Or they say that life is more like a large painting. Its dark portions seem pointless when we stand too close. But when we stand back enough to view it as a whole, we can see the contributions that even its shadows make.

Other Christians qualify the idea that God is completely loving. Some of these hold that even before they are conceived God freely chooses whom he will love and whom he will hate. Others take a more measured approach. They contend that in our time the word "love" has become so sentimental that many take for granted that it is better to feel good than to be good and to do good. Given this widespread meaning of the word "love," they contend that it is better not to apply it to God.

Yet other Christians take a hard look at the idea of divine power, recognizing that there are some things God cannot do. God cannot do that which is self-contradictory. For example, no matter how vigorous the effort, God cannot make $2 + 3 = 7$. Also, God cannot do that which is contrary to God's own moral character. An example of this is that God cannot command the torture of innocent children or compel unfaithful spouses to stop cheating.

Taken together, these three "limitations" on divine power make it less plausible to hold God unilaterally responsible for evil. Yet even if this alternative reduces the perplexity and doubt that evil causes, something that many Christians doubt, it does not eliminate them. To some extent, this challenge to Christian faith always remains.

As Christians struggle to understand the meaning of pain and suffering on the macrocosmic level, they are also confronted with many health issues that demand decisions for moral and ethical living. Being in optimum health and making wise ethical decisions that impact one's health are not only a necessity for survival and vibrant living, but also a fulfillment of the divine mandate to be a caretaker of the gifts and resources granted by God. All Christians take seriously Apostle Paul's words, "Whether you eat or drink or whatever you do, do it all for the glory of God" (1 Corinthians 10:31). We will see, however, that on some of the most talked-about and relevant health and bioethical issues of daily living, Christians are once again divided. In the paragraphs that follow, we survey five such issues – diet, procreation, abortion, stem cell research, and homosexuality.

For most Christians, the issue of diet is a very personal one. A great majority of Catholics, Protestants, and the Orthodox do not have imposed restrictions on diet – what one can consume and not. For them, the death of Jesus voided the distinction between clean and unclean meat that are found in the Old Testament and opened the avenue for a life of freedom on dietary matters as long as one's health is not injured. A minority of Christians, however, have insisted that faithful stewardship of the divine gift of health entails avoidance of food and substances that are known to have negative health consequences. Taking the original diet found in Genesis 1 literally, such Christians have advocated vegetarianism or even strict veganism as the ideal diet to follow. They have argued that human beings were created to only consume nuts, vegetables, fruits and grain, and consumption of meat and fish should be avoided to lessen pain and suffering of animals and to promote greater care for the environment. Others (especially those whose religious communities were strongly impacted by the health and societal reform movements of nineteenth-century America) have argued that alcohol has no place in a Christian's life since it is known to be a harmful substance. Most Christians, however, do not follow such restrictions and argue instead that the freedom that Christians find in the salvation offered by Jesus allows them to make individual decisions on these matters. They would oppose excessive consumption of alcohol and meat, but do not find moral or biblical arguments against moderate consumption of either.

Historically, Christians have had strong views on human sexuality. Virtually all of them agree that this part of life has two purposes. One of these is the unitive purpose (making love) and the other is the procreative purpose (making babies). It is very difficult to find Christians of any sort who object to this. Differences of conviction surface when it is asked whether it can be ethically permissible for Christian husbands and wives intentionally to separate these. At this juncture, Evangelical Protestants and Mainline Protestants tend to see things one way and Roman Catholics another, while Orthodox Christians are divided on the issue.

Roman Catholicism teaches that it is not ethically permissible for Christian husbands and wives intentionally to separate the unitive and procreative purposes of human sexual intimacy. This is one reason why it opposes sterilization and contraception. Orthodox Christians have historically agreed with Catholics on this issue, but since the 1970s they have moved toward allowing individual believers to make procreation decisions, except for abortifacient measures, which they continue to oppose strongly. Evangelical and Mainline Protestants have difficulty following Roman Catholicism's line of thought when it teaches that artificial insemination, in vitro fertilization, and surrogate gestation inherently violate the unitive purpose of sexual intimacy. They agree that every new human life should begin in loving actions, but not all of them understand why it is unloving for a Christian husband and wife to become parents by working with fully qualified medical specialists in fertility clinics.

When it comes to the issue of abortion, Evangelical Protestants, Catholics, and the Orthodox stand in sharp contrast to Mainline Protestants. The former group has taken a very restrictive position by maintaining that performing or having an abortion is ethically wrong unless it is the foreseen but not intended outcome of attempting to save the pregnant woman's life. This point needs to be emphasized because some mistakenly say that the most restrictive Christian position on abortion means that, if it is necessary to choose between the lives of the embryo or fetus and the pregnant woman, her life should be sacrificed. This is not so. That it is not so can be established by recalling that in the cases we are usually talking about, ectopic pregnancies and uterine cancers, it is often not possible to save the fetus. On the other hand, Mainline Protestants are willing to view abortion with regret but moral approval in cases like rape, incest, profound fetal malformation, and extreme maternal distress.

The considerations that inform the intra-Christian debate on abortion surface again with respect to stem cell research. A key issue, which is also intensely debated when the morality of abortion is being discussed, is the "when" question. Everyone agrees that somewhere in the process of human gestation a line must be drawn, even if it is not entirely precise, between a new human life that the state must protect and one that it need not. Christians answer this question in two primary ways. Many say that conception is the time and this precludes stem cell research on human embryos, though it certainly can continue elsewhere, as Orthodox Christians, Catholics, and Evangelical Protestants think it should. Others hold that successful implantation, not conception, is the time. This makes it possible to do stem cell research on the thousands of no longer needed embryos in fertility clinics that will otherwise be discarded. Those who draw the line at implantation do not necessarily forbid abortion from there on out; however, they hold that this decision is ethically more weighty than preventing the implantation of fertilized ova or doing research on them.

Homosexuality is another issue that divides Mainline Protestants, on the one hand, and Evangelical Protestants, Orthodox Christians, and Roman Catholics, on the other. Most in the latter group of Christians view the homosexual identity as an aberration from God's created order and condemn homosexual practice as sinful. They regard the creation of Adam and Eve and their heterosexual identity and relationship as providing a normative view of human sexuality. Their view is further buttressed by such passages as Romans 1 where Apostle Paul makes a strongly worded denunciation of male and female homosexuality as found in the Roman world. Many in the Mainline Protestant churches, however, view homosexuality either as a trait that eventually emerged in the human race as part of God's creative activity or as an aberration from the creation norm of heterosexuality yet one that does not need to be condemned – like, for example, being nearsighted or flat-footed. Both groups within Mainline Protestantism interpret the specific biblical statements on homosexuality as reflecting the cultural norms and biases of the time, thus not directly applicable in the modern era. For them, it is necessary to take into account recent scientific findings and to listen carefully to homosexuals. At the same time, there are many who belong to Mainline churches who, on this issue, agree more with the Evangelical Protestant/Roman Catholic/ Orthodox wing of Christianity. This debate explains the reason why the National Council of Churches (a coalition of Mainline churches) has declined to take a stand on same-sex marriage, for example, whereas the National Association of Evangelicals, the Roman Catholic Church, and the Orthodox Church in America have officially opposed it. Perhaps more clearly than anywhere else, on this issue we see the deep and wide chasm between at least two different ways of reading scripture, viewing reality, and interacting with important ethical issues of our time.

Death and dying

Virtually all Christians in the United States accept the two standard ways of understanding death. One of these is that death is the total and irreversible loss of circulatory (pulse) and respiratory (breath) functions. The other is that death is the irreversible loss of the functioning of the entire brain, including the stem. Though most Christians agree on the physiological meaning of death, the differences that lie among them on its theological meaning lead to different conclusions on such end-of-life bioethical issues as euthanasia and suicide.

The word "euthanasia" is an English term derived from the Greek language that literally means "good death," not "mercy killing." Deciding which kinds of death are genuinely good requires an individual or group to face two distinctions. One of these is the difference between voluntary euthanasia and non-voluntary euthanasia, the first being a death that a mentally competent patient chooses voluntarily and with adequate information.

Virtually all Christians approve of not always doing everything to keep a patient alive. They agree with the Bible that there is a time for everything, including a time to die, and that all others should respect this. About such measure – also called passive euthanasia – the consensus is overwhelming.

However, most Christians – again most Roman Catholics, Evangelical Protestants, and Orthodox Christians – oppose active euthanasia, an act of shortening the process of dying by doing something that intentionally ends a patient's life. But it is also the case that they usually look with favor upon giving the dying patient enough medicine to keep him or her comfortable even if doing this unintentionally causes the patient to die more swiftly. This is because Christian thinking has long distinguished between outcomes that are merely foreseen, on the one hand, and those that are also intended, on the other. They hold that it is ethically wrong intentionally to shorten a patient's life, but it is not necessarily ethically wrong unintentionally to shorten his or her life while intending only to relieve suffering.

Christians who favor the use of palliative care that might hasten the dying process point to three analogous situations that seem to justify their view. One of these is that surgeons foresee that they will leave scars but do not intend to do so. Likewise, oncologists foresee that the chemotherapy they administer will have uncomfortable and unsightly side effects but they do not intend this. Still further, those who apply radiation therapy foresee that they will probably damage some healthy flesh but they do not intend this. However, Mainline Protestants, who are swifter to approve active euthanasia, frequently object that the difference between outcomes that are merely foreseen and those that are also intended is a semantic quibble with no intellectual substance.

Suicide is seen with disapproval by most Christians, even though the biblical writers sometimes report that someone ended his or her own life without expressing moral approval or disapproval. Some have gone so far as to say that it is an "unpardonable sin" because it is the only one for which it is impossible to ask forgiveness. In previous generations, Christians have dishonored the bodies of those who committed suicide and denied them burial in Christian cemeteries. Few Christian groups approve of such treatment in the twenty-first century, many preferring to view one who has committed suicide as an individual who was overcome by difficulties in his or her life.

This negative attitude toward suicide is still evident in widespread Christian opposition to laws, like those in the states of Oregon and Washington, that allow doctors to give patients prescriptions for medicine with which they – the patients themselves, not the doctors – can end their own lives. Again, almost all Evangelical Protestants and Roman Catholics oppose it whereas a significant number of Mainline Protestants do not object and those who do are usually not strident.

Christians ritualize death and the grieving process in diverse ways but follow a common theme of hope and comfort. For Roman Catholics, it is important for the dying to receive the sacrament of prayer for the sick conducted by a priest in preparation for death. Once the patient dies, three rituals traditionally take place: (1) the vigil or wake at which family and friends spend prayerful time together with the deceased person; (2) a requiem mass at a church or cathedral which is led by a priest, and (3) the rite of committal where the loved one is laid to rest. Protestants typically have three events that parallel these; however, they can be less formal and traditional. Protestants often speak of separate meetings for: (1) the viewing of the deceased (though it is often not held), (2) the funeral or memorial service led by a minister or a spiritual leader and involving family members, and (3) interment at the burial site. The Orthodox Christians have a four-part process: (1) the Trisagion service (to ask God to grant rest to the departed soul), which takes place the night before the funeral service at the wake; (2) the funeral service with an open casket at an Orthodox church led by a priest; (3) burial at graveside asking God again to give rest to the soul of the deceased; and (4) *Makaria*, a "mercy meal" shared by the mourners to celebrate the life of the deceased, traditionally with fish as a sign of fasting and mourning.

While Catholics, Protestants, and the Orthodox all permit autopsies, particularly when required by law, they are divided on the practice of cremation. Orthodox churches view cremation as desecration of the body, thus funeral services with cremated remains are not allowed in Orthodox churches. Until the 1960s, Roman Catholics were of the same position, but they have since relaxed their stance, allowing for individuals and families to decide and giving permission to priests to hold funeral masses with cremated remains. Evangelical and Mainline Protestants, on the other hand, leave the issue of the disposition of the body to the patients and their families.

Conclusion

Over the last 2,000 years, Christianity has made many twists and turns while never entirely losing its own identity. At this time in the United States Christianity is a conglomerate of diverse theologies and historical expressions with Roman Catholics, Orthodox Christians, Evangelical Protestants, and Mainline Protestants aligning themselves in different ways from one issue to another. For the most part, although there are important exceptions, Catholics, Evangelical Protestants, and the Orthodox tend to represent the "conservative" wing of Christianity, while Mainline Protestants tend to occupy the "liberal" wing. This pattern is evident and persistent in the relationships between these Christian groups and health and

Table 11.1 Dos and don'ts

Dos	Don'ts
1 Remember how large and diverse Christianity is.	1 Do not act as though all religious people are ignorant.
2 Keep in mind the general bioethical tendencies of Evangelical Protestants, Roman Catholics, and Mainline Protestants.	2 Do not think that if you know what one Christian believes you know what they all believe.
3 Understand the difference between foreseen and intended consequences and why many Christians think it matters.	3 Do not tell patients that suffering is part of God's plan.
4 Enlist the help of Christian chaplains, ministers, and priests.	4 Do not override the medical choices of mentally competent, informed, and un-coerced people because of your own religious beliefs.
5 Seek mentally competent, informed, and voluntary consent.	5 Do not assume that they will eat anything offered.
6 Relieve pain and suffering.	

healing. Despite stark differences on a number of theological and bioethical issues, however, Christians are still able to find connectedness with each other through their common commitment to understanding and applying the Bible, common faith in Jesus, and mutual engagement in the world for positive transformation.

Case study

DK was a 32-year-old Amharic-speaking Eritrean refugee. He was in America ten months as a dishwasher when diagnosed with an advanced astrocytoma. The initial prognosis of many years decreased to weeks, possibly months, upon further diagnosis. Though single, DK had a support system made up of other Eritreans shaped by their Orthodox Christian religion. They believed that "God would heal DK" and insisted we do everything. This was counterintuitive to the medical team's understanding of his disease and their disposition to palliative care.

Culture and religion were an interwoven framework for DK and his support system. This framework was confusing to our medical team and it was uncomfortable to hear, "God will heal him," in the face of a terminal malignancy. The healthcare team assumed they did not fully understand the grim prognosis. DK, his support system, and eventually his mother, Gabriel, were all involved in decision making for his care, even though none of them were at his bedside. They had an accepting attitude about death, but they felt it was wrong for any person to state when it might come. That was God's work. We were to do what we do to keep DK alive and leave death and its coming to God. Only God can know if and when death would come to DK.

Differences in the definition of family emerged. DK had "cousins" all over the world and it seemed as long as they were from Eritrea, they were "cousins." DK's medical power of attorney, one Dr. Z, was an Eritrean and a practicing physician in the United States. Dr. Z acknowledged he did not know if or how he was related, but he explained that Eritreans provide support to each other when outside their native land. Community decision making was the standard and Dr. Z refused to make medical decisions without the agreement of several of DK's cousins. This was a difficult process and we hoped once his mother arrived at his bedside, things would be easier. We were wrong. She also insisted we involve his entire support system. Dr. Z acted as an advisor and educator assisting with the health-care teams' navigation amidst the unfamiliar religious and cultural beliefs.

DK was occasionally able to discuss his prognosis but his mother asked that "we allow him to die in peace." What she meant was that she did not want us to tell him that he was dying. With Dr. Z's support and guidance, we discussed with his mother the difference between medical ethics of the United States and Eritrea. He helped us bridge our differences and eventually DK and his mother were able to talk openly with the palliative care team so he fully understood that he was dying. He died comfortably with his mother at his side.

Questions for reflection

1   Are religion and culture inextricably intertwined with each other? Or can we say that there is a pure form of Christianity that can be traced back to Jesus himself?
2   Is it not a fundamental premise of medical care that patients know their diagnosis and prognosis? Should we allow families to thwart our efforts to fulfill this principle?

Glossary

Body of Christ   Either the Christian church as the continuation of the ministry of Jesus Christ or the substance of the bread after it has been changed into the body of Jesus Christ in the Mass.

Deism   Reduction of religion to what reason can establish; belief that God created the world but that now it functions on its own; partly a religious response to the European Enlightenment.

Eastern Orthodoxy   One of the three major branches of Christianity first centered in the Eastern portion of the Roman Empire but now world-wide; originally Greek in language and culture.

Evangelical Awakening   Widespread and somewhat emotional revival in eighteenth-century England and North America of Christianity; partly a religious response to the European Enlightenment.

Fundamentalism   Intensely negative reactions among twentieth-century Protestants primarily in North America against attempts to modernize Christianity; sought to get "back to basics."

Protestantism, Evangelical   More conservative Christian churches in the United States that descend from the sixteenth-century revolts against Roman Catholicism led by Martin Luther and others. Simply "Protestant" in much of Europe.

Protestant, Historically Black   African American Christian churches in the United States that descend theologically from the sixteenth-century revolts against Roman Catholicism led by Martin Luther and others.

Protestantism, Mainline   More liberal Christian churches in the United States that descend from the sixteenth-century revolts against Roman Catholicism led by Martin Luther and others.

Roman Catholicism   One of the three major branches of Christianity first centered in the Western portion of the Roman Empire but now worldwide; originally Latin in language and culture.

Sacrament   Christian ritual or practice that conveys divine grace in human life. A "visible sign of an invisible reality."

Sin   Thought, word, or deed contrary to the will of God. "Original sin" used as a theological term refers to the first sin by the first humans, Adam and Eve. The subsequent negative consequences of this original sin affect the lives of each human person.

Trinity   The only true God, who exists of one substance in three persons, in whom Christians believe.

Bibliography

Chalcedon Christology Formula (451 CE) Center for Reformed Theology and Apologetics. Available online at: www.reformed.org/documents/index.html?mainframe= www.reformed.org/documents/chalcedon.html (accessed December 21, 2008).

Edwards, J. (1959) *Religious Affections: The Works of Jonathan Edwards*, vol. 2, Smith, J. E. (ed.) New Haven: Yale University Press.

Nicene Creed (325 CE) Center for Reformed Theology and Apologetics. Available online at: www.reformed.org/documents/index.html?mainframe=www.reformed. org/documents/nicene.html (accessed December 21, 2008).

Wormald, B. (2015) *America's Changing Religious Landscape*, Pew Research Center. Available online at: www.pewforum.org/2015/05/12/americas-changing-religious-landscape (accessed June 1, 2016).

Suggested texts

Eck, D. L. (2002) *A New Religious America: How a Christian Country Has Become the World's Religiously Diverse Nation*, New York: HarperCollins.

Gausted, E. S. and Schmidt, L. (2004) *The Religious History of America*, revised edition, New York: HarperCollins.

Marty, M. (2008) *The Christian World: A Global History*, New York: Random House.

Meade, F. S. and Hill, S. S. (2007) *Handbook of Denominations*, 12th edn, Nashville: Abingdon Press.

Numbers, R. L. and Amundsen. D. W. (eds) (1986) *Caring and Curing: Health and Medicine in the Western Religious Traditions*, with a foreword by Martin E. Marty, Baltimore: The Johns Hopkins University Press.

12 Recent religious movements in America

Julius J. Nam

Christian Science
There is no life, truth, intelligence, nor substance in matter. All is infinite Mind and its infinite manifestation, for God is All-in-all. Spirit is immortal Truth; matter is mortal error. Spirit is the real and eternal; matter is the unreal and temporal. Spirit is God, and man is His image and likeness. Therefore man is not material; he is spiritual.

Mary Baker Eddy

Jehovah's Witnesses
The world is fast coming to realize that the "kingdoms of this world" are not Christlike, and that their claim to be of Christ's appointment is not unquestionable. Men are beginning to use their reasoning powers on this and similar questions; and they will act out their convictions so much more violently, as they come to realize that a deception has been practiced upon them in the name of the God of Justice and the Prince of Peace. In fact, the tendency with many is to conclude that Christianity itself is an imposition without foundation, and that, leagued with civil rulers, its aim is merely to hold in check the liberties of the masses.

Charles Taze Russell

Latter-day Saints
All who have died without a knowledge of this gospel, who would have received it if they had been permitted to tarry, shall be heirs of the celestial kingdom of God; also all that shall die henceforth without a knowledge of it, who would have received it with all their hearts, shall be heirs of that kingdom; for I, the Lord, will judge all men according to their works, according to the desire of their hearts.

Joseph Smith, Jr.

Seventh-day Adventists
As the health of invalids improves under judicious treatment, and they begin to enjoy life, they have confidence in those who have been instrumental in their restoration to health. Their hearts are filled with gratitude, and the good seed of truth will the more readily find a lodgment there and in some cases will be nourished, spring up, and bear fruit to the glory of God. One such precious soul saved will be worth more than all the means needed to establish such an institution.

Ellen G. White

Introduction

America, in the mid-nineteenth century, was a place of great religious ferment. The Second Great Awakening of the 1820s and 1830s brought a new revival in personal religion and spirituality among Protestant Christians. Protestants, who comprised the dominant majority, continued to carry the belief that America was a land of destiny with a special purpose in the world. This belief, as well as a sense of optimism and adventure that came with the founding of the new nation and the modern progress in science, technology, and industry, contributed to the flowering of new religious and social movements that sought reform in religion and society.

Each of the religious movements discussed in this chapter arose as an expression of and response to that reform impulse in nineteenth-century America. Each presented a strong, unique vision of religion and American society and demanded radical dedication to the faith and practice of the community.

Demographics

Latter-day Saints

As of 2015, the Church of Jesus Christ of Latter-day Saints reported worldwide membership of 15.6 million in more than 30,000 wards (equivalent to local congregations). The United States had the highest number of Latter-day Saints with 6.5 million. Within the United States, the western states of Utah, California, Idaho, and Arizona had the highest number – with Utah leading the way with two million. Globally, the church was active in more than 120 countries, especially in Central and South American countries, Australia, Canada, Japan, the Philippines, and the United Kingdom. Mexico and Brazil had the largest number of Latter-day Saints outside of the United States, each with about 1.3 million (Church of Jesus Christ of Latter-day Saints 2015).

Seventh-day Adventists

Within the United States, California has the highest number of Adventists with 182,000, followed by Florida, Oregon, Texas, Washington, Michigan, and Georgia (General Conference of Seventh-day Adventists 2008). As of 2014, the Seventh-day Adventist Church had 18.5 million members worldwide in 78,810 local churches. Adventists have an active church presence in 201 nations. India had the highest number of Adventists in any country with 1.5 million, with Brazil coming a close second with 1.45 million. The United States had just over 1 million (General Conference of Seventh-day Adventists 2015). Church membership was particularly strong in eastern and southern Africa, the American continents, parts of Southeast Asia, and the Indian sub-continent.

Christian Scientists

Per instructions by Mary Baker Eddy, the founder of the Church of Christ, Scientist, Christian Scientists do not publish actual membership figures. They reside in more than 130 countries, with more than 2,000 churches. Groups affiliated with the Church of Christ, Scientist, such as reading rooms, publishers, and social service enterprises as well as churches, are active in 80 countries. The churches are called branches of the "Mother Church" in Boston, Massachusetts. As of 2005, there were over 1,100 certified Christian Science practitioners (healers) listed in *Christian Science Monitor*, a daily newspaper owned by the church (First Church of Christ, Scientist 2008).

Jehovah's Witnesses

As of 2015, Jehovah's Witnesses reported worldwide membership of 8.2 million worshiping weekly in 118,016 congregations in 240 countries (Watch Tower Bible and Tract Society of Pennsylvania 2015). The United States has the highest number of Witnesses with 1.2 million, with Mexico and Brazil coming second and third with 829,523 and 794,776, respectively (Watch Tower Bible and Tract Society of Pennsylvania 2014). As with many other Christian movements, their numbers are particularly strong in Central and South American countries and Eastern Europe. Within the United States, higher concentrations of Jehovah's Witnesses are found in southern and western states (Watch Tower Bible and Tract Society of Pennsylvania 2008).

History

Latter-day Saints

The Church of Jesus Christ of Latter-day Saints (or Mormonism as popularly called) was established in April 1830 in New York by Joseph Smith (1805–1844). Smith claimed to have received visions from God who instructed him to restore the true church of Christ. An angel named Moroni directed Smith to long-hidden golden plates containing stories of God's people in the North American continent going back to 600 BCE, Jesus' revelations to Native Americans in the first century CE, and subsequent experiences of Christians in America. These golden plates were translated into English and took the name of the *Book of Mormon*. As a record of the direct revelation of Jesus, the *Book of Mormon* was considered to be of equal authority to the Bible. The restoration of the true church included acceptance of the *Book of Mormon* and Joseph Smith as a modern-day prophet.

The distinct claims of Latter-day Saints resulted in persecution of the group by Protestants, which compelled the movement to become an itinerant community. Between 1830 and 1844, Latter-day Saints moved from New York to Ohio to Missouri to Illinois, where an anti-Mormon mob killed Smith and his brother. This led them far west beyond the then-borders of the United States to what is now Utah under the leadership of Brigham Young (1801–1877), the church's second prophet – one of the tenets of the Latter-day Saint belief system being the continuing gift of prophecy in modern times. Young guided the church through the difficult early years in Utah and toward becoming the thriving global movement that it is today.

Seventh-day Adventists

The year of Joseph Smith's death, 1844, is significant for Seventh-day Adventists for a different reason. That was the predicted year of Jesus' second coming for the followers of William Miller (1782–1849). Miller interpreted the 2,300-day prophecy of Daniel 8 as pointing to the return of Jesus and the end of history on October 22, 1844. Out of what came to be known as the Great Disappointment experience of that day, a group arose who reinterpreted the prophecy in Daniel 8 as referring to the *beginning* of the final phase in earth's history and adopted the seventh-day Sabbath as the true day of worship and the end-time sign of faithfulness to God. This group, eventually known as Seventh-day Adventists, was led by James White (1821–1881) and his wife, Ellen White (1827–1915), who from 1844 claimed to receive visions from God.

In the 1840s and 1850s, Adventists' preoccupation with Christ's imminent return prevented them from engaging in active missionary work or building institutions. However, by 1863, as the church grew, Adventists organized the church formally, with their headquarters located in Battle Creek, Michigan. The formal organization of the church launched Adventists on the path of building significant publishing, educational, and medical institutions through the United States and eventually the world as they aggressively embraced missionary outreach. Significant in this process was the work of Ellen White, who shaped Adventist thought and practice through her writings on the Bible, theology, lifestyle, church work, and mission.

Christian Scientists

The Church of Christ, Scientist, was officially organized in 1879 in Lynn, Massachusetts, by Mary Baker Eddy (1821–1910). Like Joseph Smith and Ellen White, Eddy claimed to have a special experience with God and taught a distinct set of beliefs that stood in clear contrast with the dominant New England Protestantism of her time. Eddy, who grew up as a Congregationalist Christian, is said to have "discovered" Christian Science through a miraculous healing she experienced after a bad fall on the ice in February 1866. Initially, due to the severity of the fall, Eddy was thought to be dying. But after just three days of Bible reading while confined to bed, she made a dramatic recovery and "discovered" the true science of healing, particularly after her reading of Jesus' healing of a "palsied man" in Mark 9. This science, she believed, was to recognize that all reality is spiritual and to rely completely on life in the Spirit (see section "Beliefs and practices" for further clarification).

Eddy's teachings are captured in her 1875 book, which she expanded in 1883, with biblical expositions under the title *Science and Health with Key to the Scriptures*. Christian Scientists consider this book to be an inspired writing in addition to the Bible. In 1881, Eddy founded the Massachusetts Metaphysical College through which she spread her teachings on spirituality and healing. The following year, three years after the church was formally organized, the church headquarters moved from Lynn to Boston, signaling a more public phase of the community's outreach and growth. Though the teachings of Christian Science were directly at odds with the prevailing notions of knowledge, medicine, and religion, the very distinctive beliefs gave Christian Scientists a stronger and sharper identity and aided the community's international outreach.

Jehovah's Witnesses

The Jehovah's Witnesses were the last of these four groups to appear on the American religious landscape. After being involved in failed date-setting efforts for the second coming of Jesus Christ, Presbyterian-turned-Congregationalist Charles Taze Russell (1852–1916) formed his own apocalyptic Christian movement in 1879, whose primary activity was the publication of *Zion's Watch Tower and Herald of Christ's Presence*. Through this periodical, Russell advanced his own interpretation of the end-time prophecies of scripture, which included the belief that Christ had already come invisibly and his presence was increasingly being manifested in the world. Within a year, more than 30 groups formed in connection with *Zion's Watch Tower*, leading to the incorporation of the Watch Tower Bible and Tract Society in 1884. Though Russell never claimed inspiration or prophetic calling, his interpretations of scripture, including his belief that Christ's presence would reach its peak in 1914 and that World War I was the biblical Battle of Armageddon, was normative for all the members of the Watch Tower Society.

After Russell died in 1916, Joseph F. Rutherford (1869–1942) succeeded Russell as the Society's second president. It was under Rutherford's leadership that the society began calling itself Jehovah's Witnesses in 1931.

Rutherford made some revisions to Russell's interpretations, including the identification of Armageddon with World War I, and added some new predictions, including the failed claim that Old Testament patriarchs would be resurrected beginning in 1925. Another of Rutherford's innovations was resistance to governmental authority. He taught the Witnesses to resist military service and all political activity. Although the Witnesses have since experienced further failures of prophecies by their leaders and persecution from states that have not respected their conscientious objection stance toward military service, they have persevered and grown stronger through aggressive evangelistic outreach both within the US and throughout the world.

Beliefs and practices

General

Latter-day Saints

As the full name of their church indicates, Latter-day Saints clearly view their movement as a Christian church. However, they see themselves as belonging to neither the Catholic, the Orthodox, nor the Protestant tradition. Rather, they present their community as an independent branch that was raised up by God as the restoration of the true church instituted by Jesus Christ in the first century CE.

At the heart of that restoration lie their distinctive teachings on scripture, the Godhead, and the church. Latter-day Saints affirm scripture as recognized by Protestants (predominantly, the King James Version). But they differ from both Protestants and Catholics in that they accept additional writings as part of the scriptural canon: *The Book of Mormon* (believed to be a revelation of Jesus Christ given to Native Americans), *Pearl of Great Price* (Joseph Smith's corrections to the King James Version and translation of other documents), and *Doctrine and Covenants* (the prophecies of Joseph Smith and all his successors down to the present). The recognition of the latter book is based on the Latter-day Saint teaching that the gift of prophecy (and the inspired authority that comes with it) continues in the present age through the prophet of the church who serves also as the president. Another key difference between Latter-day Saints and other Christians is on the understanding of the Godhead. Latter-day Saints view God the Father, his Son (Jesus Christ), and the Holy Spirit as three distinct persons. They understand Jesus to be a literal and physical son of God the Father – thus, subservient in authority to the Father. Still, like other Christian movements, they do believe in the incarnation of Jesus – that he left the spiritual realms to become a human being in flesh – and in salvation of humankind through faith in Jesus. Finally, the Latter-day Saint conviction that their movement is the restoration of the true church of

Jesus Christ at the end of earth's history (hence, "Latter-day" Saints) leads them to hold that the ordinances of their church have unique efficacy in the world that is to come. They believe that to reach the highest degree of salvation, or exaltation, one must participate in the "saving ordinances" of their church, including particular washings, anointing, and celestial marriage, which, on earth, is available only in the church's temple.

Seventh-day Adventists

Unlike Latter-day Saints, Adventists view themselves as belonging to the family of Protestant churches and adhere to the great Reformation principles of the supreme authority of the Bible, salvation by grace and faith in Jesus Christ, and the priesthood of all believers (the idea that each believer can approach God directly and that each has a divine calling to minister to the world). They also agree with the historic Christian teachings on the Trinity, the divine-human nature of Jesus, and the importance of the church community as a manifestation of the invisible "Body of Christ."

At the same time, they hold some beliefs that distinguish them from other Protestant bodies. Among them are the teachings on Jesus' work in the heavenly sanctuary and the end-time, the Sabbath, and the gift of prophecy. When the Millerite expectation of Jesus' second coming on October 22, 1844, ended in what has come to be known as the Great Disappointment, a small group of would-be Seventh-day Adventists banded together to introduce a new interpretation claiming that Jesus, instead of returning to the earth, entered the Most Holy Place (the divine throne room) of the heavenly temple. This, they believed, was the beginning of the final period in earth's history during which Jesus was engaged in the investigation of all of humanity – dead and alive – to vindicate the true character of God and make the final determination of those eligible for eternal life. Since then, this belief has gone through several refinements, but Adventists remain officially committed to the belief that the final period in earth's history began in 1844 and that Jesus is engaged in a special end-time work in heaven. While this "sanctuary doctrine" was being developed, another of Adventism's distinctives was also being formulated – the recovery of the seventh-day Sabbath. Early Adventists believed that the "Christian Sabbath" of Sunday represented departure from the biblical Sabbath of both the Old and the New Testaments, which, they preached, was the same as the seventh-day Sabbath of the Jews. They further taught – and Adventists continue to teach – that the keeping of the Sabbath has special significance as a test of loyalty in the final days of earth's history. Finally, like Latter-day Saints, Adventists believe that the biblical gift of prophecy has continued throughout Christian history and was given to Ellen White, one of the founders of the church. Though she never claimed to be a "prophet" and the acceptance of her writings is not a condition for membership in the Adventist church, White is widely considered to have received the prophetic gift and her writings, though subservient in authority to scripture, hold a special value in the life of the community.

Christian Scientists

Like Latter-day Saints, Christian Science does not see itself as belonging to any of the historic streams of Christianity. Rather, it claims to be a separate, unique phenomenon that recovers the healing power of God and the truth about reality. They agree with other Christians that the Bible is God's revelation and that Jesus who was the divine son of God was born of virgin birth and was resurrected after being crucified. They, however, do not read the Bible literally, but primarily metaphorically and allegorically, resulting in a theological system very different from most other Christian bodies.

Apart from their views on sin, death, metaphysics, and healing, which are discussed later in this chapter, other areas of uniqueness for Christian Science include their views on God the Father and Jesus Christ. Christian Scientists used the term "Trinity" to refer to the three-person Godhead of the Father, Christ, and the Holy Spirit, but their conception of the three is unique. For them, God is both a father and a mother figure who is different from Christ, the spiritual manifestation of God. God is simultaneously identifiable as the distinct "Divine Mind" and all of reality. Christ, then, is a manifestation of God which came to physical reality and became Jesus the human. Jesus was able to heal and perform other miracles because of Christ's manifestation of God in and through him. However, Christian Science distinguishes Jesus from Christ, teaching that the former was merely the bodily existence displaying Christ. Through this Jesus, though, God pointed to the true nature of reality – that it is spiritual – and the power available to all human beings from God through prayer.

Jehovah's Witnesses

The belief system of Jehovah's Witnesses shares many characteristics found among the three other movements discussed in this chapter. They also view themselves as the restorers of the true understanding of the Christian ideals, yet hold some very distinct ideas that separate them from all other groups within Christianity. Like Latter-day Saints, Adventists, and many other Christians, they view the Bible as God's Word and read it more or less literally, and they believe in salvation through faith in Jesus Christ who died for the sins of humanity. Jehovah's Witnesses agree with Latter-day Saints and Adventists in the belief that the end of history is near and that their movement has been gifted with a special message for the end-time. Along with Latter-day Saints and Christian Scientists, they reject the historic Christian understanding of the Trinity. Instead, they, like Latter-day Saints, take literally the biblical expression of Jesus Christ as the "son" of

God and see him as a divine figure subordinate in authority to God the Father. Also, much like Latter-day Saints and Christian Scientists, they do not see themselves as following a particular branch of Christianity, but as constituting a unique, independent, and the only true stream. Hence, they find it their mission and calling to convert the entire world to their movement.

Some distinguishing features of Jehovah's Witnesses' beliefs include the particular use of the name Jehovah, their view on the two classes of salvation, and their relationship with society and governmental authorities. They have found it important to emphasize their allegiance to Jehovah, the English version of God's name found in Exodus 3:14, hence placing it in their name. They believe that there will be two classes of saved – the heavenly class consisting of the 144,000 (as referred to in the Book of Revelation) and the earthly class who will receive eternal life after Jesus' second coming and live on earth. The Witnesses believe that God began gathering the special group of 144,000 from 2,000 years ago and that process ended in 1914, as taught by Charles Taze Russell. Thus, the only hope for those who live today is to join the earthly class. Another notable distinctive belief and practice of Jehovah's Witnesses is their neutral stance in the political arena. This stance arises out of their commitment to God's kingdom rather than earthly governments. Though they pay taxes and obey the laws of the land, they do not believe in participating in politics and serving in the military (even when drafted) as these activities do not allow them to maintain neutrality in times of conflict. Furthermore, they do not salute the flag or observe national holidays and other holidays of religious origin as, they believe, these can easily lead to excessive nationalism and propagation of false religious beliefs (since many of the religious holidays are of mixed, multi-religious origin).

Health and bioethical issues

While Latter-day Saints, Seventh-day Adventists, Christian Scientists, and Jehovah's Witnesses all base their beliefs on the Bible and confess Jesus Christ as their Lord much like most other Christians, they have distinct beliefs and practices on health that set them apart. Still, all four of these groups share the general Christian commitment to physical, emotional, and relational health, based on the biblical teaching that the human body is a "temple of the Holy Spirit" (1 Corinthians 6:19). It is on the specific interpretation and application of the Bible's teachings on health that they differ.

Latter-day Saints

Latter-day Saints believe that it is a religious duty to take good care of the physical body with which the spirit is united during life on earth. The body is considered a gift from God which plays an important part in one's "eternal progression," the process of growth toward perfection that began before birth and will continue forever. What happens to the body and how one takes care of the body have consequences that go beyond this life. They also teach that the family is the basic unit of the church and the basis for a righteous, holy life. Every person is viewed as a child of heavenly as well as human parents, as each in his or her premortal life was created by the Heavenly Father and Heavenly Mother and part of the eternal family. Through birth, the person who was in the spirit state is joined with a physical body so that one can go through the process of eternal progression and reach higher levels in the spiritual realms.

Based on this belief, devout Latter-day Saints consider consumption of alcohol, tobacco, coffee, tea, and narcotics as violations of God's health laws. Coffee and tea are not to be taken due to their caffeine content, which can be habit-forming. Latter-day Saints tend to avoid other caffeinated drinks, such as cola products, as they too can be habit-forming, though technically this latter injunction is not considered to be mandatory. As for the dietary concerns, Latter-day Saints believe that all will become vegetarians during the Millennium, the 1,000-year period of peace which will commence with the second coming of Jesus, but none are required to be vegetarians. Still, meat is to be eaten sparingly, and all are encouraged to consume vegetables, fruits, and grains. These teachings are based on "Word of Wisdom," a section of *Doctrine and Covenants*, the 1835 book by Joseph Smith, which is considered part of scripture by Latter-day Saints.

On a number of sexual and biomedical issues, Latter-day Saints hold conservative positions. They believe that sexual activity, including passionate kissing, outside of marriage is wrong. Although until 1890 they believed in and practiced polygamy, they teach monogamy – union of a man and a woman – as the only norm for marriage. They consider homosexuality a sinful condition and condemn its practice as unbiblical and unnatural. They oppose abortion, considering it a violation of the commandment not to kill (Exodus 20:13). Only in extraordinary circumstances can abortion be permitted – in cases of rape, incest, grave danger to the mother's life or health, and fatal defect in the fetus. In such situations, they are instructed to consult church leaders and give time for prayerful consideration before deciding on abortion. Latter-day Saints do not approve of artificial insemination except within a marriage relationship. They also discourage using genetic materials other than the husband's or the wife's. At the same time, this decision is ultimately left up to the couple. On the issue of birth control, Latter-day Saints do not have a mandatory rule for all. However, because of the importance they place on family and the responsibility to bear children, they have historically encouraged child bearing and discouraged permanent birth control methods such as vasectomies, tied fallopian tubes, and premature hysterectomies. But, in the end, the decision remains with the couple.

Seventh-day Adventists

"The health message," as referred to by Seventh-day Adventists, is a major component of their beliefs and practices. This teaching began to develop soon after the church's formal organization in 1863 after Ellen White claimed to receive a vision about the importance of physical health and its connection to the mind and spirit. In 1865, White reported another vision in which she was given the message to start a medical institution. This resulted in the first Adventist healthcare institution, the first of hundreds to follow.

Helped by White, Adventists soon made the link between their health teachings and their belief about the human nature. Unlike most other Christians, Adventists hold that human beings are indivisible, organic unions of the body, mind, and spirit. Rejecting the view that human nature is composed of the body and the soul, they believe that the human person is the soul who completely ceases to exist at the time of death (without the "soul" going to heaven or hell). Because they view human nature as a composite of the body, mind, and spirit, they have found a deeper reason to value wholeness – harmonious development of the physical, mental, and spiritual health – even claiming that this experience of wholeness is part of one's preparation for the second coming of Christ.

In practical terms, the Adventist emphasis on health has led the church to promote healthy diet and lifestyle. Adventists condemn the use of alcohol, tobacco, and narcotics and recommend against caffeinated drinks such as coffee and tea. They teach vegetarianism as the recommended dietary norm and refrain from unclean meat as described in the Old Testament book Leviticus, chapter 11. There, "unclean meat" is the meat of animals that do not have split hoofs or chew the cud and the fish and seafood that do not have fins and scales. At the same time, dietary decisions are ultimately left up to the individual. Adventists are active in smoking-cessation efforts, prevention and treatment of alcohol use, and promotion of vegetarianism through their global network of healthcare institutions.

Like Latter-day Saints, Adventists tend to lean toward the conservative side of the social spectrum on issues dealing with sexuality and biomedical ethics. Adventists do not condone premarital or extramarital sexual activity, though the extent to which one engages in expressions of affection prior to intercourse is left up to the individual. Because they hold that appropriate sexual intimacy can occur only between a man and a woman in a marital relationship, Adventists do not accept homosexual romantic relationships or practices as legitimate. Abortion is unacceptable when it is performed as a means of birth control. Understanding it to be tragic, there are occasions, such as rape and/or incest, when abortion is thought to be justifiable. Adventists leave the final decision to the woman. Decisions on birth control and various methods of assisted human reproduction, including artificial insemination, are left up to the individuals involved.

Christian Scientists

Given their root experience in the healing of Mary Baker Eddy, health and healing are part of the core beliefs of Christian Scientists. They hold that God and all of creation are good and spiritual – being non-material. They believe that the material reality is illusory and that true spiritual understanding leads to the recognition of the spiritual reality as the only true reality. Christian Scientists believe that it was through such realization that Eddy received healing and that all seekers of spiritual truth can experience healing and liberation from sickness.

Christian Scientists' belief about reality leads them to prefer prayer as the primary, if not exclusive, means of healing and therefore refrain from using modern medicine. Prayer for them is a method, or "science," through which one experiences awakening to the true nature of reality and connection with the healing power that is available in that reality. Important in this process are the church's recognized Christian Scientist Practitioners, who provide spiritual treatment through prayer and use of scripture and Eddy's *Science and Health with Key to the Scriptures*. This treatment is covered by some insurance companies and recognized by the United States government as a legitimate medical expense. While Christian Scientists give strong preference to prayer and spiritual healing, they are not forbidden to receive medical services. Many do go to hospitals for births, broken bones, or treatment for emergency care due to accidents, but others choose to rely exclusively on spiritual healing. When they do seek medical services, they tend to avoid the use of drugs and pain relief as these are understood to have a negative impact on the spiritual nature of the person. However, the specific decisions on when or whether to seek medical care belong to the patients and their families.

As for the specific lifestyle and bioethical decisions, Christian Scientists tend to be conservative, though they leave many decisions to individuals. Marriage is generally viewed as that between a man and a woman, and premarital and extramarital sexual activities are not condoned. Christian Scientists do not have an official position on homosexuality, abortion, birth control, or assisted human reproduction. They do not follow a particular diet, although they tend to abstain from alcohol, tobacco, and other stimulating and intoxicating substances.

Jehovah's Witnesses

As part of their commitment to the body as the temple of the Holy Spirit, Jehovah's Witnesses value healthful living in all areas of life. As with Seventh-day Adventists, Jehovah's Witnesses hold the view that the human soul is mortal and integrated with the body. Thus, they believe that the soul dies at the time of death and becomes nothing – until the time of the second coming of Jesus, who will resurrect the saints to eternal life. But, unlike Seventh-day Adventists, Jehovah's Witnesses have not made this belief an essential part of their mission and global health work.

One key distinctive mark of Jehovah's Witnesses' teachings about health focuses on human blood. They take literally such biblical passages as Leviticus 17:10, 11, where God condemns eating of meat that has not had the blood removed (kosher meat) and Acts 15:28 where Christians are instructed to abstain from blood. This is so because blood, according to the Bible, represents life. Acceptance of these passages has led Witnesses to rule out consumption, storage, and transfusion of blood or any of its parts at all times – even when threatened by death. They are also discouraged from receiving organ transplantation since others' blood may be introduced to their bodies through the organs. This belief regarding blood has stimulated Witnesses to seek alternatives to medical procedures that involve blood transfusions, leading to innovations in bloodless surgery techniques. The church's Hospital Information Services promotes greater public awareness of bloodless surgery and facilitates such procedures for its members with cooperative medical institutions.

As with the other three groups, Jehovah's Witnesses hold conservative views on sexuality and many lifestyle issues. They view marriage as taking place only between a man and a woman and condemn premarital and extramarital sex and homosexuality as sinful. They also condemn abortion and assisted reproductive measures that involve semen or eggs of individuals other than the couple involved. As for dietary concerns, Jehovah's Witnesses do not have particular restrictions, except for consumption of meat with blood in it. They abstain from certain substances such as tobacco and narcotics, but alcoholic and caffeinated beverages are acceptable as long as individuals consume them in moderation.

Disease

Latter-day Saints, Seventh-day Adventists, and Jehovah's Witnesses view diseases and illnesses as consequences of sin. Based upon passages in the Old Testament, they view sin as having entered the universe through archangel Lucifer's rebellion against God. After his rebellion, Lucifer is also known as Satan or the Devil, who tempted and deceived Adam and Eve, the first human beings created by God and placed in the paradisiacal Garden of Eden. Adam and Eve were indeed deceived and their "fall" is how sin entered the world. Sin is defined as disobedience and rebellion against God and it has resulted in pain, suffering, further disobedience, broken relationships and environment, and ultimately death.

The three traditions commonly hold that sin has created physical and environmental conditions leading to physical and psychological dysfunctions, diseases, and illnesses. They also hold that the intemperate choices that individuals make – which are also consequences of the sinful condition of the world – contribute to sickness of all types. They do not distinguish between physical and mental illnesses, but view both in physical and spiritual terms. These illnesses have natural, physiological causes that can be managed or overcome through modern medicine, though Jehovah's Witnesses notably take exception to the transfusion and storage of blood. They do not see utilization of modern medicine and naturalistic scientific understanding and practices as running counter to their belief in the spiritual dimension of human suffering. Prayer for healing does accompany the employment of modern healthcare, though individuals in each of the three traditions recognize that ultimate healing will only be possible when the fundamental cause of sickness – the sinful, corrupted condition of the world – is overcome at the time of the second coming of Jesus. At that time, Jesus will eradicate sin from the earth and bring about a perfect, sinless, disease-free state of being.

Christian Scientists, on the other hand, do not locate the cause of human suffering in one historical event, whether it is Lucifer's rebellion or the fall of Adam and Eve. In fact, they do not take the biblical story of creation and fall as historical accounts. They only take the story of Adam and Eve as allegories that teach the nature of sin, which they define as fear and ignorance. Diseases and illnesses, according to Christian Scientists, are the result of human ignorance about the truth nature of God, or the Divine Mind, and reality. They teach that God loves every individual and that true reality is spiritual and non-material. They assert that the physicality and sickness as typically experienced by human beings are illusory. Once individuals abandon false understandings of God and reality and experience re-orientation of thought toward the true reality that is spiritual, sickness will disappear, even in this life. As noted already, due to such a strong belief in the spiritual nature of healing, Christian Scientists generally avoid modern medical care, including blood transfusion, organ transplantation, and drugs that affect the mind, such as pain medication.

Death and dying

Latter-day Saints

Latter-day Saints' belief in life after death allows them to accept it as the passage to the next phase of life, though they neither seek it nor embrace it openly. Upon death, all will proceed to the spirit world until the day of Jesus' second coming and resurrection of these spirits. At that time, all will be assigned to different levels of God's kingdom according to their actions and affiliations while on earth. Opportunities for accepting Jesus will be given to spirits even at that time and those who do accept him will join the process of "eternal progression" toward the status of divinity. Satan, his devils, and those who persist in rebellion against God will be thrown into "outer darkness" as eternal punishment.

Latter-day Saints are encouraged to bury their dead in the ground in keeping with the biblical practice of returning "dust to dust." However, if the local law requires, other practices such as cremation are allowed. Latter-day Saints who have received the "Temple Endowment," a particular privilege to take part in temple services, are dressed in a temple garment before burial – with the women of the Relief Society dressing women and men who have been ordained as priests dressing men. Typically, a funeral and/or graveside service presided by a bishop or his representative precedes the burial. The burial may include the dedication of the grave as a holy resting place until the day of resurrection. The grave then becomes a sacred site for the family of the deceased. Suicide is denounced as wrong, but Latter-day Saints reserve the ultimate judgment to God. They generally condemn physician-assisted suicide and active euthanasia, but give room for allowing patients to pass away rather than keeping them alive in vegetative or extremely painful and miserable conditions in the final stages of terminal illnesses. In such dire situations, the decision is left to the patients and their families and caregivers. Autopsies may be performed, if required by law and/or consented by the family of the deceased.

Seventh-day Adventists

While Seventh-day Adventists view death as an abhorrent consequence of sin, they emphasize the hope that they hold for resurrection at the time of Jesus' second coming. As noted already, Adventists believe that one goes neither to heaven nor hell after death, but the soul (i.e., the person) dies and ceases to exist. Their hope lies completely in God's power and promise of resurrection. The wicked, who persist in rebellion against God until the time of death, are expected to receive the final judgment of complete non-existence, which constitutes the Adventist understanding of hell. While they believe heaven to be a literal place, Adventists do not believe that hell represents an actual location but a metaphor for eternal non-existence.

Adventists do not have a prescribed ritual connected with death, though they typically hold funeral and burial services to celebrate the life of the deceased and encourage the loved ones in the knowledge that she/he rests in peaceful sleep until the coming of the Lord. These services are similar to most Protestant funeral rites; they involve singing of hymns, reading of scripture, pastoral homilies, tributes by family and friends, and prayers. Both burial and cremation are acceptable, and autopsies may be performed. While efforts to prolong life are positively viewed by Adventists, they do not oppose cessation of life support when signs of consciousness and of the possibility for recovery have ceased. They oppose suicide, assisted suicide, and active euthanasia, though the church's response in such difficult situations is one of ministry and support, rather than condemnation.

Christian Scientists

Death for Christian Scientists is an illusion. It, along with decay and sickness in life, is a result of erroneous understanding of God and the spiritual nature of reality. Thus, with proper understanding and insight, it can be overcome. When one does die, Christian Scientists do not consider the event as necessarily a tragedy as it represents release into the mental, spiritual state of existence where the individual's consciousness will continue in its quest for purer understanding of God and reality. Christian Scientists believe that this process of "purification" will continue forever with neither reward nor punishment awaiting the end of this life or future transitions in phases of existence.

Christian Scientists do not have a pre-determined method of marking death or preparing for death. Given their particular view toward modern medicine, it would be important to ascertain the exact wishes of the patients and their families nearing death as to how they wish to receive medical care, if at all. The church does not have an official position on euthanasia or assisted suicide, though suicide in general is considered to be against the divine principle of life. All decisions – including the method of disposition of the body – are left to the dying and their families. Christian Scientists hold memorial services typically at home or the funeral home. Since they do not have ordained clergy, family members or recognized leaders of the local Christian Science community may preside.

Jehovah's Witnesses

Jehovah's Witnesses view death, hell, and the nature of afterlife in the same way as Seventh-day Adventists. They also believe that death and hell mean complete non-existence and that the righteous will be resurrected (i.e., given new existence) at the time of Jesus' second coming and live forever with God experiencing the reward of eternal life.

Care for the dying and disposition of the dead are largely left to the individuals and their families. While they do not believe that scripture requires indefinite life support, Jehovah's Witnesses believe in maximizing the length and quality of life. Thus, they oppose suicide, assisted suicide, and active euthanasia. Autopsies of the deceased are accepted, as are cremation and burial, depending on the wishes of the families. No particular funeral services are prescribed for Jehovah's Witnesses, though typically a "memorial talk" will be held at the Witnesses' Kingdom Hall or a funeral home, followed by a graveside service. These services consist of a homily by a community leader based on scripture and prayers of comfort for the families.

Conclusion

Though Latter-day Saints, Seventh-day Adventists, Christian Scientists, and Jehovah's Witnesses share many important commonalities with other

Christian traditions, such as Catholicism and mainline and evangelical Protestant groups, they bear some prominent beliefs and practices on health, human nature, and death that set them apart. The distinguishing features result from each group's different interpretations of scripture's teachings on health, sin, human nature, and reality, though the four do share a generally similar outlook on sexual morality and importance of right, healthful living. Each in its own way represents a response to the challenges that the advancement of modern science posed to nineteenth-century America. Latter-day Saints and Seventh-day Adventists showed great openness to the healing methods of modern science and allowed the best of science to inform their health practices. Jehovah's Witnesses generally followed the same path, though they could not embrace modern science as openly as the former two due to the literal reading of scripture's teachings on blood. On the other hand, Christian Science represents the strongest exception taken to modern science, denying its premise of viewing reality as material. In a different way, though, the four movements represent the common nineteen-century American openness to bold experimentation with new interpretations of scripture and new ways of being Christian – a tradition that has continued in manifold ways throughout the twentieth century and into the twenty-first.

Table 12.1 Dos and don'ts: Latter-day Saints

Dos	Don'ts
1 Be respectful of the patient's dietary specifications (no caffeine). 2 Involve the family in decision making. 3 Ask if the patient wishes to see a Latter-day Saint leader.	1 Do not speak condescendingly of the patient's or Latter-day Saints' view on diet. 2 The preferred name of the group is "Latter-day Saint," rather than Mormon, though the latter is not an offensive term.

Table 12.2 Dos and don'ts: Seventh-day Adventists

Dos	Don'ts
1 Be respectful of the patient's dietary specifications (often no meat or fish). 2 Be respectful of Sabbath considerations. 3 Facilitate the patient's wish to use a more natural means to the degree that it is possible. 4 Facilitate the patient's desire for prayer and anointing by an Adventist pastor or elder.	1 Do not speak condescendingly of the patient's or Adventists' view on diet and Sabbath-keeping.

Table 12.3 Dos and don'ts: Christian Scientists

Dos	Don'ts
1 Explain fully and clearly the physiological effects and implications of each procedure. 2 Ask to what degree the patient wishes to receive medical care and drugs and respect his/her right of refusal. 3 Find out what arrangements the patient and his/her family has made for the dying. 4 Help locate a Christian Science practitioner for prayers of healing. 5 Allow time for personal prayer.	1 Do not speak condescendingly of the patient's or Christian Scientists' suspicion toward medical care. 2 Do not insist on specific care that the patient is uncomfortable with. 3 Do not make any medical decisions, even simple ones, without explaining everything fully.

Table 12.4 Dos and don'ts: Jehovah's Witnesses

Dos	Don'ts
1 Respect the patient's desire to avoid blood transfusion and storage. 2 Explain fully and clearly how the blood will be used and disposed of when it is drawn. 3 Work with the Hospital Information Services of Jehovah's Witnesses' Watch Tower Society if bloodless surgery is an option. 4 Be sensitive to the fact that Jehovah's Witnesses do not involve themselves in politics or celebrate holidays, including birthdays.	1 Do not speak condescendingly of the patient's or Jehovah's Witnesses' view on blood. 2 Do not make any medical decisions, even simple ones, without explaining everything fully.

Case study: Mormonism

A student in my clinical ethics course approached me after class to ask for advice regarding what she should do with the frozen sperm of her deceased son. She explained that ten years' prior she was married and she and her husband were active members in the Church of Jesus Christ of Latter-day Saints (LDS). Shortly after their only son's sixteenth birthday they had received the devastating news that their son had leukemia. Assuming that treatments would cure their son but leave him sterile, they collected sperm samples that their son would presumably use when he was older.

Unfortunately, their son passed away before his seventeenth birthday and within another year the husband and wife divorced. She had become an atheist and he had left the LDS Church in favor of a fundamentalist sect of Mormonism. Their son's sperm samples were not considered during the divorce negotiations. A decade passed. During this time the husband had remarried but suffered testicular cancer rendering him sterile. He could not have his own children and his only remaining option for promoting his own genetic line was to utilize his deceased son's sperm. Within his fundamentalist sect, he found a 19-year-old woman who was willing to be posthumously married to his deceased son and be inseminated with the boy's sperm, thus bearing his grandchild.

My student's former husband approached her about ownership of the sperm. As they had divorced in California, they had equal ownership over the sperm. She was horrified by his proposed plan and she wanted their son's sperm destroyed. He argued that as a Mormon their son would want his line continued for the sake of having his own family in heaven.

My student refused to grant him use of the sperm. The man refused to give his permission to have the sperm destroyed. He wished to move forward and had retained legal counsel. The woman argued that her son, a believing member of the LDS church, would not have believed in a posthumous marriage or in fathering a child after his own death, especially not with a young woman who was willing to enter into such an unorthodox arrangement. The man argued that his son would have followed him in faith to the fundamentalist belief system and would have wanted it to ensure his eternal happiness.

Questions for reflection

1   Assuming lawyers were able to gain ownership/custody on behalf of one of their clients, what should a fertility specialist do? Is it right to use the sperm of a long-dead minor to create life?
2   Can we speculate as to what the deceased young man would have wanted spiritually? Is this sort of arrangement religiously acceptable in such groups?
3   Is this really a case for lawyers or is there some religious/ethical approach that can help resolve the issue?
4   Can we question the mental competency of the 19-year-old woman willing to be inseminated with the deceased 16-year-old's sperm?

Glossary

Latter-day Saints

Book of Mormon   A book believed to be a revelation of Jesus Christ that contains stories of God's people in North America throughout the centuries.

Endowment   Ritual consisting of symbolic acts and covenants that is performed in a Latter-day Saint temple.

Joseph Smith (1805–1844)   The founder and first prophet of the Church of Jesus Christ of Latter-day Saints.

Temple Recommend   A certificate given to Latter-day Saints by church leadership for entrance to the temple. It is given only after the member is able to show worthiness by answering a series of questions.

Seventh-day Adventists

Ellen White (1827–1915)   One of the co-founders of the Seventh-day Adventist Church.

Great Disappointment   A term used to describe what took place on October 22, 1844, among those who awaited the return of Jesus Christ that day.

Health message   Adventist teaching about the connection between the body, mind, and spirit and the importance of complete wholeness as part of one's preparation for the second coming of Christ.

Vegetarianism   Adventists recommend vegetarianism as the ideal dietary choice. It stems from their emphasis on health as part of the call to a life of wholeness.

Christian Scientists

Divine Mind   Another name for God. Used very often due to Christian Scientists' emphasis on the mental and the spiritual as the only reality.

Mary Baker Eddy (1821–1910)   The founder of Christian Science.

Practitioners   Individuals who practice healing through prayer according to the principles of Christian Science. Qualified practitioners are typically listed in the *Christian Science Journal* and www.spirituality.com.

Science and Health   A book written by Maker Baker Eddy and published originally in 1875 and expanded in 1883 with "Key to the Scriptures." Considered an inspired book that stands on equal footing with the Bible, it provides a description of the principles of Christian Science.

Jehovah's Witnesses

Bloodless surgery   A method of surgery without the use of another person's blood; some may choose to use their own blood in a bloodless surgery.

Charles Taze Russell (1852–1916)   Founder of the Jehovah's Witnesses movement.

Kingdom Hall   Meeting place of the Jehovah's Witnesses, the external appearance of which is similar to a modest Christian church yet without any of the typical external symbols.

Watch Tower Society   The central administrative organization of Jehovah's Witnesses.

Bibliography

Church of Jesus Christ of Latter-day Saints (2015) "Statistical Report 2015." Available online at: www.lds.org/general-conference/2016/04/statistical-report-2015?lang=eng (accessed June 13, 2016).

First Church of Christ, Scientist (2008) "About the Church of Christ, Scientist." Available online at: www.tfccs.com/aboutthechurch.jhtml (accessed December 14, 2008).

General Conference of Seventh-day Adventists (2008) "145th Annual Statistical Report – 2007." Available online at: www.adventistarchives.org/docs/ASR/asr2007.pdf (accessed December 14, 2008).

General Conference of Seventh-day Adventists (2015) "151st Annual Statistical Report – 2015." Available online at: http://documents.adventistarchives.org/Statistics/ASR/ASR2015.pdf (accessed June 13, 2016).

Watch Tower Bible and Tract Society of Pennsylvania (2008) "Statistics: 2007 Report of Jehovah's Witnesses Worldwide." Available online at: www.watchtower.org/e/statistics/worldwide_report.htm (accessed December 14, 2008).

Watch Tower Bible and Tract Society of Pennsylvania (2014) "Jehovah's Witnesses Reach Membership Milestones." Available online at: www.jw.org/en/jehovahs-witnesses/activities/ministry/how-many-jehovahs-witnesses-2014/ (accessed June 13, 2016).

Watch Tower Bible and Tract Society of Pennsylvania (2015) "How Many of Jehovah's Witnesses Are There Worldwide?" Available online at: www.jw.org/en/jehovahs-witnesses/faq/how-many-jw-members/#?insight[search_id]=95febd96-8c84-4035-9fe6-a5c057ceaf0a (accessed June 13, 2016).

Suggested texts

General

Albanese, C. L. (2007) *America: Religions and Religion*, 4th edn, Belmont, CA: Thomson.

Miller, T. (1995) *America's Alternative Religions*, 2nd edn, Albany: State University of New York Press.

Moore, R. L. (1986) *Religious Outsiders and the Making of Americans*, New York: Oxford University Press.

Neusner, J. (ed.) (2003) *World Religions in America: An Introduction*, 3rd edn, Louisville, KY: Westminster John Knox.

Latter-day Saints

Bush, L. E. Jr. (1993) *Health and Medicine among the Latter-day Saints: Science, Sense and Scripture*, New York: Crossroad.
Church of Jesus Christ of Latter-day Saints (1948) *The Book of Mormon: An Account Written by the Hand of Mormon upon Plates Taken from the Plates of Nephi*, Salt Lake City: The Church of Jesus Christ of Latter-day Saints.

Seventh-day Adventists

Knight, G. R. (2004) *A Brief History of Seventh-day Adventists*, Washington, DC: Review and Herald.
White, E. G. (1905) *Ministry of Healing*, Mountain View: Pacific Press.

Christian Scientists

Eddy, M. B. (2000) *Science and Health with Key to the Scriptures*, Boston: First Church of Christ, Scientist.
Knee, S. E. (1994) *Christian Science in the Age of Mary Baker Eddy*, Westport, CT: Greenwood Press.

Jehovah's Witnesses

Bergman, J. (1984) *Jehovah's Witnesses and Kindred Groups: A Historical Compendium and Bibliography*, New York: Garland.
Watch Tower Bible and Tract Society of Pennsylvania (2005) *What Does the Bible Really Teach?* New York: Watch Tower Bible and Tract Society of Pennsylvania.

Conclusion

There is a tendency in Western medicine to search for physical explanations of sickness and diseases – to find the right virus, to locate the tumor, to search for the specific neuron. And the quest goes on for the cure and the best treatment. These chapters exploring health and disease from the perspectives of world religions remind us that illness is a universal human experience. Illness affects the physical, mental, emotional, and spiritual realities of all human persons. Conversely, we learn from the wisdom of these religions that the way we see reality, the way we interpret events, and the way we connect with Divinity can impact the way we experience health and illness.

Healthcare providers have come to the important realization that the way one lives out religious beliefs influences profoundly the experience of sickness and the process of healing. We have learned the possible variations in the way people may interpret cancer, kidney disease, heart failure, and many other diseases, and the way belief systems impact health and the treatment process. This understanding of the role of interpretation of sickness and health necessitates careful consideration in treating patients from various faith traditions because it is ultimately the patients' religious understanding of the meaning in life that defines health and wellness for them. The lack of understanding of patients' belief systems can lead to deterioration of their health because it can potentially create internal conflicts that generate negative thoughts, emotions, and spiritual experiences.

This understanding of the role that religion plays in healthcare generates a different sort of question for healthcare providers to ponder – questions regarding the validity of various faith traditions and the different approaches they can (and ought to) take toward other religions. Initially, there are two options: open and closed. One can either be open to the possibility that true and genuine religious beliefs and experiences are possible in more than one religion or be closed to that possibility. For those who belong to the latter group, there is only one valid religion – their own. For them, other religions may offer specific teachings that are valid, truthful, and useful, but no other constitutes a valid religious *system*.

On the other hand, those who are open to seeing other traditions as valid religious systems have further questions to consider. Are all religions equally valid? Are there degrees of validity? Are there any objective criteria with which to evaluate religions? If so, what are they and who sets these criteria? If not, are all evaluations of religions ultimately subjective? For some, while they recognize that other religions can offer valid pathways to the Divine, they view their own as the definitive religion that offers the best and clearest religious teaching and experience. As for other religions, they tend to accord varying degrees of validity depending on the religions' proximity to their own.

Others view all religions as more or less equally valid. Some among them accord validity to all religions as long as they adhere to certain general criteria, such as recognition of the Divine and practice of distinct rituals and ethical behaviors. Others in this camp believe that it is impossible to establish any meaningful objective criteria for a valid religion and leave the judgment to individual decisions.

Yet others seek to bridge these various approaches by acknowledging *without judgment* the various religious ways of being, living, and believing, while holding firmly to one's own religious tradition. They tend to stress dialogue among religions and mutual learning among the followers of the world's religions – including those who do not identify with a specific religion and even agnostics and atheists.

Regardless of the approach we take as individuals or as religious communities on other religions, the attitude that has motivated the editors and authors of this book is one of understanding and respect. In an increasingly shrinking world where religions, denominations, sects, and groups interface with one another daily, it is important – regardless of how one views other religions – to understand and respect who the followers of the world's great religions are, where they live, what their history has been, what they believe and experience in life, how they view health and disease, and how they confront the profoundly vexing question of death and what lies beyond. Understanding and respect do not equal agreement or even appreciation. But they lead to more informed interactions that lead to friendlier neighborhoods, healthier societies, and a more peaceful world – and in your professional sphere, a more compassionate patient care.

In addition to the manner with which we interact with those of other religious traditions, we trust that in your work as a healthcare practitioner your education about the religions in this book will enhance your professionalism and compassion. As noted in the preface, when individual practitioners and entire facilities pay attention to the religious practices and needs of patients, everyone is benefited. The individual patient's healing encounter is enhanced, the practitioner experiences a more fulfilling encounter with the patient, and the facility itself incurs greater respect and credibility in the local community it serves.

As Western medical science evolves along its technological path, it will likely also learn to be more open and appreciative of other, less technical, means of dealing with illness. These less technical, more traditional, and deeply religious methods of addressing human illness should enhance

Western medicine rather than clash with it. We hope that clashes can be avoided as we learn more about the traditional and religious methods of handling illness. Yet we also want to urge practitioners not to simply accept each and every religious or traditional method. Some methods may in fact harm patients rather than help them. But it is only a discerning practitioner, one who has taken the effort to learn of the Other, who will be able to address the healing encounter with balance and equanimity.

Like the healing enterprise, religion is not staid, religion and its traditions are ever evolving, always adjusting to the cultures they encounter and help to shape. Thus it is that many of the issues addressed in this text are relatively new and troublesome things for religion to deal with. The advance of medical technology brings the difficult questions of life-sustaining healthcare, reproductive assistance, abortion, and even diet. This list can be lengthened but the point is, just as was noted in the introduction to the text, religion and culture are ever and always in an elaborate and complex interaction with each other. Culture and religion continually modify each other and so it should be no surprise that medicine and religion will do exactly the same thing. While the questions of life and death remain the realm of faith and religion, medical technologies and cultural acceptance of these technologies change the way we discuss life and death in religious circles. Take, for instance, the notion that life begins at the moment of conception. Religion has – through its non-scientific lens – traditionally taken this moment to be when a woman gets pregnant. Well, in this day and age when every moment, that is every nano-second, is studied by medical scientists in the effort to understand, enhance, and protect human conception, the "moment of conception" becomes something far more important and definitive. When a religious leader stands and speaks of the moment of conception and a medical researcher stands and uses the same phrase, we see that the two may be speaking of the same event with quite different emphasis. And thus science and religion interact and influence each other.

The same can be said of the matter of death. Prior to the technical capability to measure activity in the brain, a person was considered dead when the heart stopped pumping and the person stopped breathing. Religion has always had something to say about death and yet, in this day when machines and drugs can keep these functions active, we wrestle with what it means to be "brain dead." Religion continues to be relevant even in the face of shifting scientific definitions of life and death.

Finally, our introductory chapter author, Ernest J. Bursey, suggested that the readers of this text would benefit from the purposeful encounter with someone of a different religion. He included three case summaries about persons in healthcare who had encountered the Other and learned something in the process. Have you done the same over the course of reading this text? We certainly agree with Bursey and want to cap off this conclusion with a reminder that, in engaging the Other, you and your healthcare practice will be enhanced and enriched.

Index

Page numbers in *italics* denote tables.

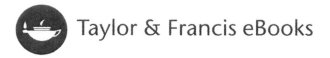